For Carol

The
Perfection
of
Hope

A
Soul
Transformed
by Critical Illness

Elizabeth Simpson

Macfarlane Walter & Ross
Toronto

Copyright © 1997 by Elizabeth Simpson

Macfarlane Walter & Ross
37A Hazelton Avenue
Toronto, Canada M5R 2E3

Canadian Cataloguing in Publication Data
Simpson, Elizabeth, 1941–
The perfection of hope: a soul transformed by critical illness

ISBN 1-55199-008-3

1. Simpson, Elizabeth, 1941- -Health.
2. Spiritual formation.
3. Cancer – Religious aspects.
4. Lungs – Cancer – Patients – Canada – Biography. I. Title.

RC280.L8S55 1997   362.1'9699424'0092   C97-930930-1

Printed and bound in Canada

Macfarlane Walter & Ross acknowledges
the support of the Canada Council for the Arts and
the Ontario Arts Council for its publishing program.

For patients everywhere
and for those who give them hope

Hope is the thing with feathers
That perches in the soul.

EMILY DICKINSON

I believe hope can surprise you.
It can survive the odds against it, all sorts of
contradictions, and certainly any skeptic's
rationale of relying on proof through fact.

AMY TAN
The Hundred Secret Senses

Contents

Acknowledgments

I did not write this book alone. The emotional support and practical help of my husband, Noel Schacter, cheered me up, calmed me down, and enabled me to complete the lengthy process with my health intact. My unique writing club of three women who have met over ten years, Rona Murray, Alisa Gordaneer, and myself, gave me perspective from two generations other than my own – one with the wisdom of age, the other with the exuberance of youth. As well, each chapter was initially discussed with two encouraging friends, Jennifer Hyndman and Trudy Pallan. I am grateful too that a significant person from the family of each patient I mention agreed to read the relevant pages before their publication. *The Globe and Mail, The Saanich Review,* and *Homemaker's Magazine* published modified versions of four chapters. In addition, I wish to thank my colleagues at Camosun College for their encouragement. Most valuable, however, was Gary Ross, my editor, in combination with Wendy Thomas. Gary kept faith when I wavered and, with his eye for refinement and organization, he added precision and clarity to my writing. Together these people became the book ends that upheld my dream of sharing my story.

1

Seeds of Hope

Hope seldom lives alone. It depends on spiritual connectedness and the goodwill of others. To move from terror to tranquillity, the heart of the comforted must enter into an exchange with the heart of the comforter. The hand of compassion sculpts the health of the willing patient. By reaching outside the narrow cycle of our own lives, each of us becomes a participant, allowing this cycle to welcome change and to include death without inviting it. The stories in this book explore the possibility that hope may be a powerful medicine in regaining and maintaining health or, when that is no longer possible, a source of inspiration that enables a dying person to leave behind the sweet scent of courage to soothe and inspire those who have dwelled in the circle of loss.

Hope is a gift and a discipline. It illuminates and transcends the moment; it overflows with expectation and dances on the promise of fulfillment. Like Pandora's box, the life of the cancer patient may seem at first to brim with misfortune and misgiving, making it hard to wrestle hope from despair. But I have discovered with my own cancer that the soul has muscle of its own, muscle that needs exertion to stay supple and responsive. Once the recovering patient has dug far enough down to find hope, she will discover a moment of truth. Each of us reaches a point when we must create our own personal myths to live by, our own sense of what will be unleashed in the effort to find sanctuary on earth or an inspirational passage into death. I have found that the larger my awareness becomes, the denser my sphere of reference. I no longer have to look too far behind or too far ahead to find meaning that uplifts me. Smiling eyes, a voice of solace, one's hand in another's – these moments create a shield between despair and hope.

Cancer has made me aware that my presence adds its own drop of meaning to the galaxy and that my small accomplishments can reverberate for others, as theirs do for me. This knowledge is one of the gifts that a dangerous illness has brought me; its concomitant self-esteem is also, I suspect, a necessary ingredient for survival. Recognition and purpose form two lower rungs that a patient must climb to inch up the ladder toward well-being and productivity. I found that after I and the people close to me had acknowledged the realities of my disease, had accepted and accommodated them, only then could I get back into the community of human exchange. As one dear friend said of the metamorphosis that has come with my diagnosis, *If you live through this ordeal, it will be the best thing that ever happened to you.*

And I *have* lived, keenly, for two eventful years since that day in December 1994 when my biopsies proved true the radiologist's warnings of a possible neoplasm. I had no idea what the word meant until I looked into my doctor's face: cancer, and an especially difficult cancer at that. Since that time the days have grown long and voluptuous, with precious moments of forgetting that I was ever ill or am now in remission, as other cancer patients assured me would happen. The stunning recognition of my own mortality (rather than simply the mortality of others) has allowed me to break through the wall of habit that once separated me from the uniqueness of each day, and to find my center again.

This crucial homecoming reminds me of one of my final conversations with my mother in the early 1980s, when I was in my early forties and she was beginning to have premonitions of her own death. We sat at my dinner table chatting over tea; she made a comment that seemed unconnected to the flow of our conversation. *Things will happen for you again,* she said. *What made you say that?* I asked. She looked into my face as into a mirror: *Your eyes are sad.* So seldom had she offered an opinion unasked, especially on the topic of sorrow, that I felt obliged to explain. *It's hard thinking of you being unwell again, and what that means to* – She interrupted: *It's not that,* and gently but abruptly changed the conversation.

I had no idea back then that she had sensed how much I had changed in the lonely years of façades. Later, after her death, a divorce freed me to be myself again. But I realize now that she saw, as mothers do, the weight of unhappiness I had grown accustomed to carrying. Cancer forced me to leave that past behind, to peek out from behind my mask and, eventually, to trust that a new love was more than illusion. As long as I safeguarded myself against pain by denying myself pleasure, I remained partially numb.

Alternative therapies played a role in leading me to the core of my being. I became stable enough to examine the nature of being a cancer patient and hence to write this book. Most complementary treatments encourage patients to concentrate on simple day-to-day plans and surprises, since these moments matter more than yesterday's mistakes or tomorrow's ambitions. They also teach that energies spent on the creative arts are never wasted. When I was a child, my father used to say, *If you put your pennies in the pot, you'll soon have a dollar.* As a cancer patient, I finally translated his words into the metaphor he intended and found my life enormously enriched. I spent a portion of my recovery time, for example, writing stories that I am now able to share. And there are other treasures not within our control, but within our power to enjoy. The promise of morning, the privacy of rain, the stillness of snow – these cannot be measured any more than the trust in a child's eyes can be weighed. Seeing the moment as a gift has become for me the elixir that turns past and future into the gold of daily hopefulness.

I began my journey on Valentine's Day of 1995, after radical surgery, with the acceptance that my lung cancer was inoperable. In the aftermath of chemotherapy and radiation, I understood that I would have to help myself toward health. Over time, and within the warm circle of other people's generosity and expertise, I designed my own Valentine, flying not only on Cupid's wing but also on the wing of the dove. In spite of having cancer and therefore being, as my naturopath said, at the end of pathology, I began a romance with life, an infatuation with the idea of making peace with myself in the here and now. I did not know then that I would be struck hard enough by Cupid's arrow to remarry, but I did know that I had to move into my remaining life. Once begun, the process seemed a natural, even desirable one, a kernel of blessing within a terrible illness.

When I was a girl, my father often told me to beware the number thirteen. I always cheeked him back, repeating what a teacher had told me: superstition grows from ignorance. I had not yet learned that we are all largely ignorant about the major forces of life: love and loss, earthquakes and ozone, sickness and health. My father would have opposed my operation date of February 13, but he was gone by the time I faced the decision. Although the date seemed ominous, I knew that operating rooms and surgeons have long waiting lists. And for the literal life of me I would not have admitted to superstition. I decided that since I would be undergoing risky surgery, the risky number was companionable in an ironic way, or so I told those around me.

Just as I inherited a genetic propensity for cancer from my mother (although no lung cancer had touched my extended family), I inherited from my father, orphaned in his youth, an ancient dread that the impossible can happen. After my diagnosis, however, I began to coddle the idea that the impossible could mean good things as well as bad. Perhaps there is truth in the idea that we find what we look for.

At first, afloat on an ocean of medical techno-babble, I discovered that serenity and openness took considerable exertion of will. When I woke from surgery, I felt overwhelmed by the unchangeable truth that cancer was clinging to my heart, just as my personal sorrows had done before it. It occurred to me that this beating organ tells a story of more than science and scissors. I needed spiritual wisdom to coax my body into enduring and responding to radical treatment. I had a sense too of needing to compensate for the power I had given the negative parts of my life by hanging onto them. Massage, acupuncture, yoga, and naturopathy gentled me along the path to letting go.

When people hear the word *cancer,* their hearts pump to a new rhythm. It matters little whether the disease is wrapped around the upper end of the torso or the lower, the brain or the femur. As I was cast into my new role as the less-than-healthy woman, my pride suffered from the realization that I was not as self-sustaining as I had thought. Yet I began to realize that I was far more self-sustaining than I had been before my illusion of control dissolved. This seemingly small shift led me to ponder rather than grasp, to be flexible rather than frozen, to negotiate through the unchangeable and complex realities of existence rather than battling them or growing apathetic. In response to these changes came a warmth of affection from others that drew me back into a sense of well-being I had not known for more than a decade.

My father had combined a respect for both the God of the Presbyterian Church, who seemed a bit unforgiving and egocentric to me, and the gods of chance, who appeared to shake down good luck and bad as mindlessly as we shake salt and pepper onto our baked potatoes. I wondered how I had sinned profoundly enough to be given one of the worst of God's maladies, or how I had insulted the gods in a manner so crass that they had played the nasty trick of giving me a choice of surgery or no, a choice that even a committee of specialists could not get right. Initially I felt upset and defensive about my dilemma, to say nothing of the consequent pain of a split torso. But then I remembered my mother musing that she had *deserved* her illness, and my telling her that justice had no authority in the arms of disease. Eventually, empowered by the opportunity to use my new awareness, I opened up, as my ribs had temporarily done, to a discovery. I created hope from the idea that a surgeon's first-hand peek at my lung could divulge far more than x-rays ever would.

The doctor, no longer dependent solely on the vague light and shadow of x-rays, was able to pass on highly accurate information to the cancer clinic oncologists before they began their radiation and chemotherapy. Together the medical team offered, if not the promise of cure, at least the best treatments that science has

discovered to put a lung cancer patient into remission. The word
remission may not have the same clear bell tones as *cure* does, but it
seems a world away from *terminal*.

Like everyone else, I live in an unknown time zone; but my
allotment is always up for review, and I get edgy some days. When
this happens, I call to mind the comforting words of my therapists
and the memory of my former father-in-law, Gart. Healers talk of
spiritual energy and strength of purpose. These beliefs allow for a
uniqueness that Gart exemplified in his own way. He was diagnosed
with a serious throat cancer in his early fifties which metastasized
shortly after a horrendous car accident in his early eighties. He did
not despair for the interim thirty years, by waiting for the inevitable.

To survive in a meaningful way, I had to confess to a very real
need to exercise not only my body but also my imagination. I had
thought of cultural events as pastimes that come after the serious
work of earning my daily bread and keeping my house in order.
I began, however, to acknowledge further value in an afternoon
with a compelling book and a handmade quilt to buffer me against
a spiritual winter, beeswax candles at dinner to rest my eyes after a
day on the computer, or the gentle encouragement of family and
friends to keep me in the now. These became the daily bread and
safe haven of the soul. Once my torso had mended sufficiently,
I returned to attending ballet, opera, and drama with heightened
interest. My imagination seemed no longer numb and I allowed
myself to leap the realities of my wounded body, to join symboli-
cally with the dancer who pirouetted, or the singer who caused the
heart to stutter, or actors who made the audience weep and laugh.
These pleasures soothed tense muscles and deepened the breath of
hope. They came to form a portion of my life's essence rather than
an escape from it. Even when I look into the awesome face of

death, I imagine I can escape its grimness by a final act of grace – an imaginary leap into the stars while dancing to a music that astounds the galaxies, all the while whispering the most alluring words that ever spilled from soul to sense.

The day after my surgery, I sobbed with a passion of frustration and disappointment I had not experienced since it rained on my eighth birthday. I fell asleep to awake an altered person. Later I learned that complementary therapists define the lungs as holding tanks for more than air. They are storehouses for grief. Tears, according to my acupuncturist, Elena, could assist time in washing away the crimes against self that I clutched in my breast; but I had not been able to cry for many years. I had been too busy keeping my head to tend my heart. I had yet to learn that the term *breakdown* relates to more than nerves. The tissues of my body suffered, as well, in their irreplaceable home. In the months after my treatments, a surge of longing overwhelmed me, a wistfulness about tomorrow. But this future is a cautionary tale, created by a sometimes frightened woman who has realized that hope is a gift rather than a birthright, a discipline rather than an accessory, and that it depends on allowing the tears to ebb and flow with the tides of daily fortune.

I attempt in this book to share these fortunes and tragedies, as well as the abundance of fear and humor that comes with cancer. Fear visits me each time I have to return to the clinic or hospital for a checkup. Sometimes the occasion brings a retrospective humor that soothes the memory into palatable form. In December 1996, for instance, I again had to face the measure of myself, this time in the domain of laboratory technicians. My general practitioner requested a pulmonary test to determine the extent of damage inflicted on my lungs by the treatments that had arrested my cancer. After the technician brisked through the agenda, I realized I would have to be a rocket scientist and pulmonary gymnast to follow her instructions. My reluctance and her frustration increased steadily as she coaxed me into an airless glass booth where, behind a closed door, I was to sit on a stool with a plastic clothespin on my nose and a mask over my mouth and breath *normally*, while I listened to her rapid-fire instructions through a speaker.

After I had run through the test enough times to allow for an average calculation of my performance level, she asked me to pant like a dog. Having lived with a collie and then an Airedale for a total of thirty years, I cottoned on immediately. But shortly into the job, I could see the technician's disappointment. She demonstrated for me. I failed again. After three attempts, I noticed that she was panting like a Chihuahua whereas I was panting like a St. Bernard. With a quick change of my image for the word *dog,* I was able to mimic her. She then asked me to blow out a mock candle. With a device similar to a snorkeler's mouthpiece jammed between my lips and my hands pressed to my cheeks, I was to blow into a tube and raise a platform inside a glass shoe box. *No!* she said, as I blew my best. It took me a while to realize that I was blowing as I do at the candles on our dining-room table, expelling just enough air to keep wax and spit from patterning the tablecloth. She wanted me to blow as though a psychopath were tracking me by candlelight in a dark tunnel. Once I had finished blowing out the imaginary candle, I was to continue expelling air, shoulders drawn forward and down, down, down, breath easing out, head lolling toward my chest with a slow curvature of the spine, crumpling inward. The posture reminded me of that moment in marriage when one realizes that an irritant has become an irreconcilable difference. *Relax!* she hissed in my ear, and my tension increased. *Oh dear,* she remarked when she calculated my score.

At the end of the session, she looked at my file and expressed surprise: *Something's happened to you since your previous tests two years ago.* Yes, I agreed, resisting the desire to suggest that medical people should read a patient's file in advance. *It's true, something's happened to me. I had cancer, surgery, chemotherapy, and radiation.* She looked shocked: *Oh! You were burned!* I hadn't thought of it that way, although the truth of it hit home like a missile. *You mean the radiation?* I asked. *Burned,* she nodded, and I pondered the horror of her accuracy. When I left the laboratory, she called after me. *Good luck,* she said, shaking her head. I went home with the distinct impression that the scar tissue in my lung resembled a bomb site.

After a long walk, I realized I would have to dig deep to re-establish my optimism. Some lines from Pat Barker helped. In her book *Regeneration,* she wrote that "the early stages of change or cure may mimic deterioration. Cut a chrysalis open, and you will find a rotting caterpillar. What you will never find is the mythical creature, half caterpillar, half butterfly, a fit emblem of the human soul. . . . No, the process of transformation consists almost entirely of decay." I imagined beginning my task of regeneration with a damaged lobe, but proceeding to health nonetheless.

At the end of the week, I went to my general practitioner, Bill Cavers, prepared to do whatever was necessary to make this regeneration come about. He astonished me with his evaluation: I would never get back the elasticity I had lost with treatment; I would always take twice as long as people my age to recapture my breath after exertion. This doctor is talented in the art of feel-good metaphors. He explained my difficult circumstances by sending me home airborne. He likened me to a Royal Air Force fighter in World War I: So many got shot, so few came back alive, *but those who did make it, made it 100 percent.* I had my work cut out for me, then. I was simply responsible for surviving in the *now*, making do with my 43 percent ability to exhale until I was home-free on my airstrip of well-being. For the moment, I had only to avoid getting shot down by the enemy — metastasis.

My naturopath, Bruce, was quick to support the idea that, although pulmonary fibrosis suggests severe damage to the lung tissue (an aftermath of scar tissue), and that it may begin disintegration, regeneration is also possible with conscious nurturing. My acupuncturist, Elena, reminded me to think of the possibility of success. She said, for example, that the belief that severed nerve cords in the spine could never regenerate was, as we spoke, being refuted by work on our ally, the white rat.

In this book I try to share, as well, the shock of dealing with a new body once treatments are over and the routine of life has resumed. One of the strangest things about my illness is having to learn all over again in adulthood the capacity of my customary body that, except for a few extra pounds and less tautness of skin, looks pretty much as it has all my adult life. Such changes usually come slowly, allowing the ego and expectations to adjust. Not so with surgery that marks the skin, and therapies that scar the organs. For example, I had always taken the act of exhaling for granted. If I tried not to exhale, as I did to stop hiccupping, I failed. Exhaling had always seemed impossible to avoid except perhaps in shock or anger. Now I had to realize that I was not doing enough of it, and that its significance had to do with emptying the lungs of moisture and toxins and with making room for fresh air. A healthy pulmonary sac is not one that harbors bacterial sludge.

Apparently my pulmonary housecleaning was not up to snuff and I would have to give it all the tender loving care I could muster, puffing out a little farther with each yoga stretch, returning to the conservatory to resume the singing lessons that I had let go with my diagnosis, and keeping my exercise at whatever level I found possible without pain.

This revelation coincided with the arrival of painters, carpenters, and floor sanders Noel and I had hired to renew the den. We had been sidelined for a while by my illness, but eventually I had resurfaced, written a magazine article, and decided to plunge into the task of moving hundreds of dusty books to the basement and coping with my tonsils' aversion to fumes. In my eagerness I had thought autumn would be a perfect time to acquire fourteen maple shelves holding thoroughly vacuumed and alphabetized Canadian literature books, set against saffron walls and glistening wooden floors. My study began to change into the place I had imagined, but my swollen throat, stinging eyes, and aching head responded daily to the chemicals in the paint and varnish and to the sawdust that lingered in the air. I had considered this renovation a sign of my growing success as a writer, but it was proving instead to be a sign of my forgetting the needs of my body. I realized that the planning stage of renovations had been as different from the doing as reading a prescription is from swallowing medicine.

During these slip-ups, when I cannot help but wonder how long I will survive, I need to renew my sense of purpose, to make the ordinary chores of life seem worthwhile. Sometimes it's hard to resist being stopped in my daily tracks when I contemplate the permanent ravages of cancer treatments, and I forget to feel grateful for the simple and precious gift of life. I have less bargaining power now, and my sense of self-worth dips and rises as I adjust to the change.

I want assurances that I am being healed by the unique efforts of generous people, and, especially, that one of those people is me.

Where can a person in remission, with the Sword of Damocles hanging over her, seek dependable joy? How can a cancer veteran feel needed rather than needy, exude a sense of fun instead of doom? How can those who have looked on the face of death achieve the wisdom to think less on the final breath of life and more on the act of breathing? One morning, as I contemplated these questions, I absent-mindedly moved my bare foot to nestle in the fur of my loyal old Airedale, Chance. When my skin touched the hardwood floor, I realized that I had slipped into the past and was feeling the dog's presence through our habitual connection rather than her energy. After more than sixteen years of companionship, she had been dead almost a year. Her end had come shortly after my remission had stabilized; her ashes still waited to be sprinkled along the path we had walked each day.

Much is written on the well-being that dogs bring to people's lives. British and American studies have shown the benefits of pets for ailing patients or visits from animals for those suffering pain or apathy in homes for the handicapped or aged. In the Western world, the dog has become a member of the family, a four-legged medication to lower blood pressure. In Paris, for example, dogs seem at times to outnumber people. I wondered as my foot wandered if the time had come to seek out a new canine companion who would demand that I live at least fifteen more years as my part of the bargain. Having a dog would mean long daily walks like the ones I had taken with Chance during my recovery but had recently begun swapping for trips to the weight room and speed-walks on the treadmill. It would also mean the luxury of knowing that love can be as constant as the tides and as nonjudgmental as the moon. As well, it would mean living in the realm of gratitude and tail-wagging praise in exchange for keeping the chow bowl full and the heart's door open, as dogs so nimbly enable their owners to do.

And so I began a search to find again the energy that my Airedale and my collie took away with them when their long lives were over. A new puppy brought me face-to-face with the extremes of total chaos and sweet serenity (from her jumping into her freshly filled water dish to her small snores and yelping dreams that rise up from under my desk). An old experience renewed has caused me to think on the fact of serenity and that people praise each other for being intelligent, athletic, or generous, but seldom for being emotionally balanced. We hear people saying, *Gosh you're clever!* and *How do you stay so fit?* or *Thanks for your help!* But who hears anyone say, *Such balance! It's wonderful to be around.* These days, tranquillity has become central to my search for health. I try to retain my yoga master's advice that it's up to the individual to take her lessons into the world, to create a working balance on our own. Marie, a mother of five, with her noticeable intelligence, unblemished beauty, and French-Canadian accent, teaches us how to flex both our limbs and our spirits as she shares her knowledge of postures and chants before sending us home with limber spines and renewed energy.

Serenity helps too in defeating one of cancer's partners in crime – exhaustion. The psychiatrist who serves my community as a vitamin expert gave me a bit of advice as I left his office to find a health store and buy the bottles of organic vitality he had suggested for assisting me through treatments and recovery. He warned against getting tired. This seemed an attainable goal, but moderation and naps in a desperate world are not easy habits to accommodate. Over the past two years, I have developed a keen awareness of my energies, of when they are teetering off the edge. If I find myself drawn into the fray of others' demands or my own distress, I seek out my alternative therapists, who soothe the tensions of my soul that translate to my body. I have had to change my concept of how much I can accomplish in my lifetime. I used to dread the idea of retirement; I now hope to *live* to retire. I have simply had to grow attentive to my limitations at an earlier age than I had imagined. Cancer seems to have been my body's cry for a pause in the chaos, a time to search out harmonious balance.

For me harmony can be found wherever nature offers her gifts, and I suspect this is true for most people who seek to calm themselves after illness. Although I have visited many places, I have lived on the West Coast of Canada for more than two decades. Before that, I lived in only three other areas for an extended time – the prairie, where I was born and raised, immersed in its astonishing seasons; Massachusetts, where I learned to love the ocean, the intellectual buzz, and the blue-blood charm; and the Okanagan Valley, where slow summer days and abundant orchards sought out the child in me. None surpasses the West Coast with its snow-tipped mountains, deep forests, and endless shoreline. Its power speaks to primal longings and seems to heal even as it threatens.

One morning in the autumn of 1996, my eyes moved from the monotony of an unchanging computer screen to a stack of ungraded papers to the chaos of an untidy house. In the dull November light, I had lost the energy to sustain my private world through writing stories, preparing lecture notes, or keeping my home fires burning. I realized that thinking back on the end of robust friendship was making me sorrowful rather than accepting. Cancer. Grading. Dampness. My soul felt like a soggy bagel. I had forgotten how to feel grateful to be writing a book, or proud to be back teaching, or happy to be waking to the morning no matter what the weather.

To nudge myself out of lethargy, I bundled up against the damp and opened the door. The gods of sky and earth seemed to agree with my decision: the moment I turned the knob, the sun popped out, a magical array of autumn colors threading through the mist and reflecting off puddles. By the time I reached the end of the street, a team of jocks had pounced on the day from a nearby bed and breakfast. These men were obviously feeling their oats with the weather's change. One fellow had crossed to the park and begun parting company with his sweat pants. He bent over with his bare behind pointing upward, toward a large, leafless tree. *Bet he'll move if I moon him,* he said. His remark made no sense until I looked up in the direction his backside pointed. At the top of a bare branch, the neighborhood eagle had come back for his annual perch over the city as he does each November and December. The eagle waited there for his mate to join him. Every year people come to watch them in their stillness or to see them display their wing spans when they take flight. The eagle steadfastly ignored the mortal macho. *I think he prefers his female,* I called out.

Across the intersection, I turned onto a path that leads morning walkers along the ocean front. A rainbow arched across the sky, one end on the water while the other disappeared into the distant trees. The park had become a children's story that spoke of happiness in that time of year when we least expect it. As I moved toward the purple, pink, and blue archway and it played its rainbow trick of seeming to move with me, other strollers grew animated: *I wish I could get my hands on that pot of gold,* a dapper old man quipped as he turned to walk down the slippery steps to the beach. *Your eyes are the pot of gold,* an elderly woman replied. I wasn't sure whether she meant that his eyes looked golden to her or that his eyesight was the gift itself. A boy who had just zipped by me stopped on his Rollerblades to absorb the sky. He stood beside two women who leaned on their canes, necks craned in the direction of the eagle. *Describe it to us,* one of them said to the boy. *We can't see that far anymore.*

I was reminded of the day I had exclaimed over a passing pod of Orcas in the strait. The woman standing nearest me, whom I passed each morning, her little sausage dog and my enormous Airedale circling each other as though they had just met, asked if I would describe what I saw because she could no longer distinguish the killer whales from the waves. I had walked home that morning with the realization that the hope chest of old age is filled with memories stored from earlier years, and that today is the day to begin filling that chest. In time, I saw the woman without her dog; tears dripped down her cheeks when I asked the obligatory question. Later, I saw her sitting on a park bench facing the water, her face turned up toward the sun or rain. Then one day the bench was empty. Her end had seemed gradual and painless, presence merging into absence, as though the tears for her lost life had washed her away with the tide.

On the day of the rainbow, I passed a young native man sitting in the grass looking out to sea. *Did you see the rainbow?* I asked. He replied too softly for me to catch his words as he nodded toward the water. Offshore a canoe painted in the rich Haida patterns of black and red sliced through the water. A carved wooden eagle sat atop the bow, its face leaning into the journey ahead. A single native man stood in the canoe, as though following the eagle's path. It was a ceremonial canoe from the Queen Charlotte Islands. *Thank you!* I whispered.

Lungs full of air, I walked home thinking about the meaning of *breath*. Breathing had always been mindless. I never imagined that anyone would measure my exhalation and find it wanting. Neither had I really understood the two-part motion of breathing that I had taken for granted and was only now beginning to recognize. I had not even known that the body has five pulmonary lobes, three on the right and two on the left with a space for the heart. It had come as a surprise that breathing out was not the simple aftermath of breathing in, that it is an act in itself, a privilege of health. *Breathe out*, my inner voice prodded. *Further,* I coaxed my recuperating chest muscles. *You can do it!* And perhaps, with discipline and spirit, I can.

As the season of the eagle moved toward the spring equinox, I thought of the violet-green swallows I like to imagine winging in from somewhere to my back garden. During my first years in the house where I have lived since the early 1980s, the mating swallows had always heralded spring by swinging together on my clothesline. Their being together year after year seemed to tell me that my life would round itself out again, that I would survive divorce and the loss of family if I could just keep looking at this lustrous mating pair.

When Noel and I moved in together in 1993, I persuaded him to renovate *my* house into *our* home instead of moving into new territory, as he wanted us to do. We tore down the clothesline, along with the sun deck and the kitchen. No one thought to put the clothesline back up when the builders put a new cedar deck on the house. Eventually the delight of new spaces and the shock of my cancer became a part of our new lives too, and we settled into a new way of being. As one day turned into another, I began again to poke around in my flower boxes and toss seeds into the garden. The ancient apple tree blossomed and began offering its abundant fruit. The seeds took root and cosmos and poppies waved their colors in the summer breeze. Summer passed into autumn. But the violet-green swallows with their iridescent glow did not return.

From habit, I looked for them one morning and realized they had nowhere to perch, at least no clothesline on which to sway. *Please*, I encouraged Noel. *Think how wonderful our sheets and towels would smell if we let them blow in the breeze.* He promised that as soon as he had a free Saturday he would climb the tree farthest from the deck and attach the line. But the Saturdays passed and I realized that winter would soon be here, and the moment of spring would come when the mated pair would search for a summer home. *Please,* I asked again. *The violet-green swallows mean good luck for the house.* Noel told me he would have to put in a new post: *It's a bit more time-consuming than you'd think.*

Eventually I forgot about the clothesline, discouraged that I could not put it up myself and unwilling to ask again. Then one morning I raised the bedroom blind and looked out at the morning. A blue clothesline stretched from a new deck post to a sturdy poplar. It was positioned so that I could wake and watch for the birds' return. *You put up my clothesline!* I exclaimed, snuggling back into bed. *Not me*, Noel answered as he pulled the covers up to our chins. If the swallows do return to sway with us, I will again feel nature's charm. For now, I can only wait and watch. Such is the nature of hope.

Hope is the word I apply to the way I make sense of the inevitable misfortunes that come into our lives. I am in a sense *full of hope* when I find my place in the scheme of things, hope that my life will never be without meaning. The stories that follow turn on that meaning, the need for hope in various stages of cancer, for those diagnosed and those who tend them. These stories do not always have the joyful endings I may have wished, but each experience has left me richer in the knowledge of how important it is for everyone, sick or well, to realize her unique contribution to well-being. Each story has offered me a drop of understanding in the ocean of mystery that surrounds cancer.

Cancer may not be a welcome companion or a cherished friend, but it is nonetheless a visitor who will have its say. It's up to the host, then, to negotiate through the foreign terrain of this common disease. Perhaps regeneration and transformation *will* settle in on the wings of decay. Perhaps in having lost one dream of life we create another, more promising one, in the time left to us. Hope is a seed we plant in the garden of remission, keeping faith that it will root itself and bloom.

2

Robin's-Egg Blue

My parents gave their children an unusual gift. Their love for each other was palpable and lasting. It seemed to grow as they aged, always there and always appearing to surpass by a narrow margin their love for their three daughters. They did not wait in loneliness for us to arrive for random visits, as many parents do; instead, we hoped to catch them between the sundry projects they shared. In their defined roles, they worked with interdependent satisfaction to make their ever-evolving home and garden a landscape of their lives.

Perhaps they represent their time and place, having been born between the turn of the century and the Great War in settlers' homes on the Canadian prairies. My mother's childhood was an open story that we came to know during our years of growing up. She had been born of British parents who emigrated to Manitoba after their two sons were born but before they gave life to three daughters. In spite of the extraordinary physical hardships of early prairie life, my maternal grandparents gave substance to the words *fairy tale*.

When, as a woman of twenty-two, I asked my grandmother of eighty-two if she had always been happily married, she said, *Oh yes, except for the past thirteen years*. In these latter years, she had been forced to go it alone without the man who had married her as a teen-ager and remained her unabashed idol until he died. She continued this vigil until she was ninety-two, wearing his magnifiers to read the paper, sitting in his rocking chair so it did not appear empty.

My grandfather's dream had been to leave the windy homestead and set up his own shoemaker's shop on the corner of Portage and Main in Winnipeg. My grandmother loved to tell of how he went off to establish himself in the city and then, lonely for family, bicycled home sixty miles in the bitter cold of a snow-locked landscape. But he knew what he was coming home for. My grandmother loved her man, her children, her dog, and her place in their world. My grandfather was able to make his dream into a reality and eventually moved his family to Winnipeg where he supported them through his store on the famous corner. My grandparents share a grave now, beneath the elm trees that stretch across the city where they shared their successes.

In contrast, my father's life began with a tragedy that we know little about. We learned bits and pieces that we pressed our mother to tell us, always trying to manipulate her beyond the margin of solidarity with my father's privacy. His family's life on an Alberta ranch outside Medicine Hat changed in the 1920s, when a Spanish flu epidemic wiped out large numbers of Canadians, including my paternal grandmother and her youngest daughter. My grandmother was thirty-two and my aunt two years old. My grandfather became overnight a single parent, responsible for his land, his harsh job with the CPR, and his six hungry children. When he died two years later in his mid-thirties, the children were left to find their own ways among the merciless loneliness of prairie settlers.

My father was eleven when his mother died and thirteen when his father joined her; he was too old to be adopted, as his three younger sisters were, and too young to find sustaining work or marriage, as his elder brother and sister did. I suspect that my grandfather died partially from the same terminal disease that struck down my father at seventy-seven – the heartbreak that comes with loss. But I suspect as well that tuberculosis, a disease no one mentioned above a whisper in the 1920s, was the diagnosis and the reason my father never found fault with his children unless they coughed. I was raised to think that coughing was equivalent to cheeking my mother or telling a fib – immoral and disrespectful, an activity that made my father's face darken.

The night after my mother was buried, I tried to get my father to tell me what had happened between the day his own mother died and the day he met my mother at a baseball game. Instead of changing the conversation, as he usually did when he wanted to distract me, he gave me an answer with no room for argument. *It's too damn sad*, he said. Then we turned back to our task of sending thank-you notes for the many bouquets that had covered my mother's coffin. The stories he did share during my childhood were the few happy ones that had carried him through those years – the dog who returned to share their impoverished life even though an established family had offered it a home, the man who paid for my father to attend summer camp after my father had cut his lawn, the job he got at fifteen as a delivery boy for the General Steel Wares Company. All other memories seemed to begin on the day he met a young woman in a red skirt who needed coaching in the art of catching a baseball.

The problem with my parents' happiness was the seemingly unattainable ideal it established for their daughters. As our parents found solace and inspiration in the garden of their love, we learned to expect this good fortune to follow us to the altar as well. And lasting love may have been there for the taking if we had focused on strengthening the positive and accommodating the unchangeable, but by the time we each married, family values and female sweetness had lost some of their shine. Ironically, we had learned to need the kind of devotion my father provided for his wife and daughters, but we had somehow missed acquiring my mother's ability to see a man's loyalty as a well-rooted oak tree, his fragility as a precious lilac blossom, and his sexuality as a vulnerable prairie harvest.

During a post-retirement tour through the prairie provinces, my parents returned to the area around Medicine Hat. My mother wrote to me her impressions of the countryside. It was, she said, a place where "the oil rigs nodded their approval, dipping their beaks into the rich earth." Her ability to find beauty in a place where my father had suffered enormous loss was her way of gradually changing the landscape of his mind. With her strange combinations of shyness and vanity, manipulation and compliance, my mother was a savior of sorts.

When I was a child, Mother and I saved robins from the ravages of early prairie snows and from the jaws of eager felines. We put fallen baby robins in baskets hung from the clothesline. I could feel their hearts beating as I eased them onto a bed of cotton batting. Then she and I would hide to watch the mother come with a worm. I continued this practice long after I had left home. When my mother lay dying of cancer, her final words were, *Just be happy*. I was guilty of being more wordy than my mother, and I proved this in my reply: *I'll always think of you whenever I see a robin.*

One morning, not long after my diagnosis, a plump redbreast broke its neck by flying into my bedroom window. I rushed to where it had fallen under a bough of cedar. Its body quivered and its beak opened and shut as I begged it to live: *Just try, damn you!* Its head wobbled and sank to its breast. I stood outside, my hair and nightie soaked with rain, and marveled at that moment between life and death.

Unlike the ill-fated robin, my mother had proven herself able to survive seemingly insurmountable odds. Admittedly she did not try to pass through a glass window, but she did transform herself back to health after four different and serious cancers over almost thirty years. As a result of her courage and discretion, I have scant memory of her being sick, except for the time, just before her seventy-second birthday, when her fifth cancer, acute leukemia, took her beyond reach of earthly transformation.

Wing-Up. That's what my mother called her first bird, a chick among hundreds of other barnyard chicks. But this one had been trampled in the rush for warmth in the midst of a prairie winter, and it had a broken wing to prove it. My mother splintered its fragile appendage with the straightest twig she could find. When the driver came weeks later to take a truckload of young chickens from my grandparents' Manitoba homestead, their seven-year-old daughter sobbed good-bye to the one that had mended so well it was now unrecognizable to all but her eyes. The gruff driver turned out to have a heart for children, and he asked my mother what all her tears were about. As the truck drove off through the snow, she clutched the chick to her grateful breast.

Perhaps because of her early years on a homestead, Mother was able to teach me useful things beyond the kitchen and the laundry room. In my late twenties, for example, she told me that a woman's life begins at thirty. I doubt that she approved of my beginning this part of my life with a divorce, but I look back now to see some truth in her division between girls and women. It has something to do with admitting to the pleasures of the flesh. Much later, she taught me to let a freshly sharpened blade do the cutting. When, in my late thirties, I lived on a mountainside with my second husband, she came to help me settle in. As we helped my father build a closet, she encouraged me to move my arm without tension. This way, the blade and the wood, she insisted, could find their own way through the job without exhausting me. And because I had to live almost entirely by the heat of a Franklin stove, I was grateful to have learned how, with a sharp knife, to shave bits of kindling from the stack of logs my father had left behind. My mother had convinced me that fire comes from air as much as from matches, that the magic of heat begins with the spaces between wood and paper. The next year, when I failed miserably with my first garden, she told me that a plant is like any other life − it grows strong from the foundation that first gives it breath. I tapped my soil and realized that gale winds could not penetrate its hardened surface. I even learned once long ago, by watching my mother, that if I were to massage the tongue of a dying calf, it would live until morning. And because she never told me she loved me, I learned that love is in the doing.

My mother's first encounter with cancer began with a flat red blemish on her otherwise pale and porcelain skin. This barely noticeable patch made its home in the crevice between her nose and cheek. On a less clear complexion, such as the freckled faces of her three daughters, a creeping redness may have gone unnoticed. My mother was an avid gardener who had won ribbons for a Brobdingnagian carrot and a black rose (which was actually dark purple). She no doubt spent too much time under the prairie sun.

But in the late 1940s, who knew about the cumulative effects of those formidable rays? My mother's idea of a healthy life was to serve her own fresh vegetables with Sunday's roast beef and to spend holidays stretched out on a sandy beach with her husband while her children played in one of the prairie lakes. Did she use pesticides? Only when the labels assured safety. Did we wear hats? Only to church where we sat in dimly lit pews. Pesticide sprays and ultraviolet rays came with our daily ration of parental love. Just as common was the dusky chemical that rained down from small airplanes battling mosquitoes during Winnipeg's summer evenings as families perched on their front steps or rocked on their porches, inhaling the cool evening air.

As a gardener, my mother knew what to do with the diseased growth on her face. She had it scythed off to allow the rest of herself to thrive. Since she gave only a brief nod to her surgery, having to explain away her small bandage, we barely registered this momentous occasion except for noticing that she was tired and that we had to wash *her* dishes.

Mother moved through her forties to become even prettier. I remember her on Sunday mornings, making breakfast in a silken nightie that clung to her body. No cotton T-shirt for her. I figured I alone had guessed that she wore no underpants. My father, an appreciative man, adored her. They always got up at the same time each morning except on Sunday. Before church, my mother made breakfast while I crawled into her warm spot and dozed beside my father. Together we called to her from the bedroom, advising her about how many pieces of bacon we would like. With time, her cheeks had lost their paleness and taken on a rosy hue as though she were permanently blushing in anticipation of good things to come. I suspect there was truth in the idea of good things to come because my parents would closet themselves away after church, saying they wanted to *nap* uninterrupted.

The other truth behind her blush was the burden of too many red cells in her blood stream. The name for this malady is polycythemia, a cancer of the blood. To lessen her daughters' fears, she likened her blood to a soup that had grown too thick to move easily through her body. Every two months in the early 1950s, she drove her rattling Morris Minor to the hospital and underwent the medieval treatment of being bled. Afterward a nurse placed a small pillow under her head. This pillow would be exchanged for a series of larger ones until, sitting up, my mother was able to drive herself home. Generally my parents were inseparable, but Mother would never let Father accompany her on these occasions. She said he would probably have enough to do *later on*. When she arrived home, she dressed against the weather and spent long hours in her garden, harvesting strength in solitude.

In their fifties, my parents lived out a dream of returning to the birthplace of their ancestors. They hiked through the hills of Scotland and toured England, until one day my mother's abdomen swelled like a basketball. The British doctor advised her to fly home immediately. On another continent for the first time, they spent the night at Heathrow, waiting on standby, too *prairie* in their stamina to ask for special treatment. Mother's spleen had somehow worked its way into bloated exhaustion, and it had to be removed. Minus her spleen, cleanser of blood, remover of toxins, she returned to her place of healing and won a ribbon for the biggest carrot Winnipeg had ever seen.

Shortly before my father retired, my parents were suddenly

abandoned to their own resources after raising three daughters and tending to my maternal grandmother. We three daughters had scattered ourselves west of Manitoba, and my parents, except for their two-year honeymoon, were alone together for the first time in thirty-five years. Mother embarrassed me by confessing that one night, as she and my father sat reading, they simultaneously burst into tears at the prospect of never again being surrounded by family, except temporarily. My sisters and I did not know then the loneliness and fear that accompany aging and life-threatening illness. We were too busy scrambling toward our own versions of loneliness.

During this time, my mother wrote a story called "Forgive Me, I Killed a Canadian Goose." It told of a teen-age girl's encounter with an angry bird, clamped in a hunter's trap. As the rest of the flock rose from the meadow and formed an arrowhead that pointed southward, the frustrated goose flapped and called after them. Unable to free the bird, my mother had two choices: leave it to die slowly or quicken its passage. Her story, in large type on yellowing pages, dwells on the killing stone that had proved my mother a markswoman to be reckoned with. In later years, she used this same eagle eye to make grown men cry over losing yet another game of pool.

After her sixty-second birthday and my grandmother's death, my mother experienced a persistent nagging in her upper back. As her dwindling energy lessened her desire to dig in the spring earth, she longed to see her children. My sisters and I had forgotten that our mother had ever been sick. Perhaps we even wondered why other families made such a fuss over cancer. If the idea flickered that she needed us, we resolved it by remembering how adept she was at taking care of herself, how she enjoyed protecting us from her despair. Why should we interfere? After all, we were of a new generation, traveling the globe and blaming our parents for the shortcomings we discovered in ourselves.

When my younger sister, Lynne, gave birth to her first son, the doctor suggested my mother visit before her surgery. Ignoring the possibility that she was seriously ill, I worried that she might disapprove of me. Already divorced, I was living, unknown to her, with the man who would become my second husband. When I told her about my liaison, she said she was glad I was no longer alone because she would worry about me less. I promptly changed my worry to hurt because she seemed more interested in her new grandchild than in my academic papers. Without success, I had struggled for years to become pregnant by my first husband, and got no recognition for effort. I persevered with my hurt as Mother returned home to be split from navel to backbone and have her lower ribs moved aside to allow the surgeon to lift out her diseased kidney. My father phoned from Winnipeg after the operation and said, *It was what they thought*. Our parents never asked for our help, nor did they ever say the word *cancer*. Perhaps they thought it would give the disease too much power.

Once again Mother recovered. With surgery and chemotherapy behind her, she tried to persuade my father to sell the house and move to the West Coast where they could fuss over their grandchild and visit with Lynne and me. In a moment of vulnerability, he agreed to leave his prairie roots. After signing the bill of sale, however, he looked up at the prairie sky, pondered the coastal rain, and changed his mind. The new owners were convinced of the wisdom of their purchase and refused to reverse the sale. In White Rock, an hour's drive south of Vancouver, my parents carried their belongings into a cottage with a view of the ocean that would make most people sink into a comfortable chair. Not my father. He complained that it was lonely watching the sun rise and set over all that *cold* water. We rolled our eyes, making jokes about *warm* snow as he reminisced about wheat fields, the harvest moon, and the blue winter skies of Manitoba. In her spare time, my mother planted an enormous flower garden that spanned the breadth of their property. She surrounded herself with spring.

As my parents entered their seventh decade and the century moved toward its eighth, they tore down their cottage and built a sturdy home to shelter them from the winter snows that seldom fell. After listening to his neighbors and strolling the boardwalk, my father decided that the view was all right if he could just have drapes to close against the night waters. But my mother never got around to sewing drapes for the big front window. She was hemming her bathroom curtains when the phone rang to tell her that the weight loss we had barely noticed was a result of leukemia.

I drove to their door immediately and realized that, after studying the power of words for years, I did not know what to say. Trying to remember what was normal behavior, I argued with her about some political matter that both of us pretended to care about. When she left the room, my father said, *Don't argue with your mother.* I argued with him instead. *She's wrong*, I told him. He said it didn't matter anymore.

Six months later, Father and I drove into Vancouver to bring Mother home from hospital for her final Christmas. In the three hours it took to drive there, wrap her frail body in a blanket, prop her up with pillows, and bring her home, no one gave a thought to the empty fridge. We opened the door together in late afternoon, for the final time. Lighted candles on the dining table shone on a turkey, an avocado salad, and baked potatoes. Wine waited to be

31

poured into Mother's crystal glasses. I have never asked where my second husband found food on a statutory holiday or how he had learned to microwave turkey to such perfection. Perhaps I believed somehow that the magic would be lost in the knowing. But whenever I'm reminded of his wandering lusts, I remember Christmas dinner of 1983 and warmth fills my heart. When I asked my mother if she had anything to tell me, she answered true to form – with truth and brevity. *When I go, I will go quickly.*

Just before being moved to intensive care, my mother had asked that we keep our father well because he was her most important visitor. I would have faced hurricane winds to see my mother when she was moved, but I could not cross the Strait of Georgia from my home in Victoria to the hospital in Vancouver with a flu and raging cold. Not even a daughter was allowed into intensive care if she was spewing germs on those who clung to life. It was a lesson too late for the learning that the dread of losing my mother, the worry over my father's lonely future, the weight of teaching daily, and the heavy heart of marital discord wore down my immune system. My father kept up his vigil by driving twice a day on slippery winter roads between White Rock and Vancouver. He answered the call of his heart to take him to where my mother lay waiting for the end of their earthly life together. He had promised that he would be by her side to the end, and he was not one to back down on a promise.

Mother died on the last day of January while Lynne was driving Father home from their visit. The phone rang as they opened the door. The caller told my father what we all knew was coming but had somehow managed to push into the distant and vague future.

And so it was that my mother crossed over Jordan alone. My father, not one to talk of sorrow, talked of this when I was alone with him. We had just sat down for an altered version of his afternoon tea-for-two. *I told her I'd be there*, he said, his voice almost gone. *You were there*, I reminded him. *You were there for fifty years. Think about it, Dad*, I said with an authority I didn't feel.

We three daughters used our humble talents, rooted in child-hood, to say our good-byes. Joyce played the piano while the congregation sang hymns; Lynne wrote a piece of music that she performed with a friend and later recorded; I gave the eulogy. We didn't even talk through each other's performances or try to attract listeners when it was another sister's turn to shine. For once in our lives we did it for someone else. As I spoke, dry-mouthed, to the people who filled the pews, I looked down to see that my father had worn my mother's last gift. Busy to the end, she had knit him a pair of brown wool socks and a matching vest. He had managed to stuff his stockinged feet into his best shoes and wore the vest under his dark blue suit. In *The Stone Diaries*, Carol Shields named her gardening protagonist Daisy, like my mother. Both the fictional and the real Daisy were born in rural Manitoba early in the century. Shields interprets the name as *Day's Eye*. I suspect my father would have agreed; he said he missed my mother's brown smiling eyes.

At her graveside, I recited the words of the poet Al Purdy: *They had their being once and left a place to stand on.* With each passing year, those words become more meaningful to me. As I spoke at the interment, I heard the unique call of the robin. It was perched in a branch overhead, celebrating the early February sun. After Mother's funeral, elderly friends expressed their comfort in seeing that middle-aged children mourn a parent's passing. But we sisters had yet to make our words a reality, to realize that we would miss the mothering we had so often tried to escape.

The night after her funeral, I dreamed that she arrived in a shower of blossoms and took my hand. Together we floated over the neighboring houses and gardens, absorbing the extravagance of color. When we reached the water's edge, the umbilical spirit of mother and daughter was severed. In her own quiet way, though, Mother had the last word. Her garden came up in splendor the following spring, and the cactus plants she left us continued to blossom each Christmas in our separate kitchens. When we buried our father, three and a half years later, he had worn out his brown wool socks but wore his vest to rest beside her in their shared piece of earth.

Perfectionist that she was, Mother left behind three middle-aged daughters who would have difficulty matching her quiet stamina, her silky legs, her cheeky bosom. Both Joyce and Lynne had asked me privately if I thought Mother had faked her cancers. I said I didn't think so, and wondered why people tended to believe in subterfuge more quickly than in courage. When Joyce developed her own misdiagnosed cancer, she cried out for my parents. *Mom!* she called into the space of memory that had lost its sequence with morphine. *Dad!* she pleaded to the pale green walls of the hospital room. I am about the same age now as Joyce was when she died. We are daughters who did not inherit our mother's petal skin or girlish legs. Instead we inherited her vulnerability.

My mother taught me to hold with hope, to find good luck within bad, to carry on. Joyce taught me inadvertently that mid-life women are not dispensable clutter to be brushed off by the medical profession. I did not learn my sister's lesson well enough. But with the help of compassionate doctors and alternative therapists, I struggle to regain my balance and to set a new high-water mark for myself and for Lynne. Most important, remembering my father, I try not to cough.

I see a path through a wheat field, where the sky is blue and the air is dry. My mother is my age and I am thirty years younger than she is, as she was thirty years younger than her mother. From her garden, she beckons me to follow. The place we arrive at is one in which cancer can be held at bay like the weeds that threaten to overtake her flowers.

I want to ask her how she did it. I want to look into her brown and spirited eyes when she answers me. I want to tell her about the cough that turned out to be cancer. I want to tell her about the robin I could not save. I want her to forgive me.

❧ 3 ❧

Travels with a Sister

My sisters always seemed to remain the same ages. These were not specified by numerical age so much as by one's being older and the other younger than me. I was in a way buffered by their personalities, the older being stern and easily angered, the younger melodramatic and controlling. I never thought about either of them growing old. We simply moved in a trio of relative numbers.

Joyce, six years my senior, married a neighbor who was four years older than her eighteen years. In the 1950s, we all lived on the same street and drank the same water, and we all lived under the nuclear cloud that wafted from Nevada over the prairies of Manitoba. We all breathed in the pesticides that filled the summer dusk, and we all devoured the sprays that coated the vegetable garden.

Joyce and her new husband, Bob, began their family with twin births that surprised the obstetrician as well as the newlyweds. I sat at the top of the stairs and listened to my parents interviewing their prospective son-in-law: *You don't have to marry her, if you don't love her – we can bring up the baby.* First down the birth canal, Joyce had to endure our mother's idealism, a control that moderated with time, and two more daughters who were shielded by an eldest sister's trials. *I do love her*, Bob insisted. *I would have married her anyway.* Unsure of the innuendo, I was happy there would be a wedding, happy to be part of a love story that was to remain intact for a third of a century.

At nineteen, Joyce became the mother of two premature baby boys who were seriously underweight and in need of special care. Desperate with pride, she refused all help except mine. Apparently, at thirteen, I was too young to be significant, but energetic enough to be useful. I baby-sat often, cuddling the first-born, Richard, who had spent a month in an incubator and consequently missed out on the welcome given his brother, Ronald, younger by eight minutes and richer by far through daily trips to his mother's breast. Richard began as a bundle of skin and bones, wriggling inside a glass case. I loved him with the singular passion that only a budding teen-ager can feel, and I neglected Ronald with self-righteous intent. The twins began my sister's sixteen-year journey in search of a daughter.

When I was fifteen, I visited Joyce and Bob in the small prairie town of Carnduff, Saskatchewan, where he worked for an oil company. Now with three young boys, they lived in a house that had neither running water nor an electric stove. My sister filled her washing machine by carrying pails of water from a nearby pump. She kept the stove glowing and meals on the table through the scorching summer heat and into the depths of prairie winter. She told me years later that these were the happiest days of her life. Perhaps she had a sense of control, a moment in touch with needs she could answer with freshly baked bread and clean sheets flapping in the prairie wind or stiff with autumn frost. I followed her around their small wooden cottage while Gogi Grant sang to us about the restlessness of the wayward wind.

Around her fiftieth birthday, Joyce wrote me a letter, ending it with an uncharacteristically flat statement about growing tired of things that used to give her pleasure, even her children. *I never imagined feeling like this*, she said. When I had last seen her, her face had looked frozen with stamina. She seemed to carry a stone of resentment she could neither manage with grace nor cast aside. I assumed she felt cornered by middle age, sobered by the persistent drooping of flesh, awed by the deaths of our parents, and embittered by the awareness that her children had outgrown a desire for her opinions.

In the early stages of her misdiagnosed pain, shortly after she and Bob had moved to White Rock, she and I went to see the musical *Cats*. I had seen her grow teary-eyed only twice before. But when the soloist sang about smiling at the old days and being beautiful back then, Joyce swept the surrounding rows into her apron of sorrow. The power of her cancer, as yet unrecognized to all but her female soul, may have added to her sorrow over the changing nature of a woman in mid-life. She sobbed through the emotional debris of her futile anger at parents who had died before she could learn how to comfort them and at a body that had become an enemy and a stranger. The song ends with a request. The singer asks to be spiritually touched, emotionally linked, and promises that those who reach out to touch her will know happiness.

A year after this deluge of tears, the pain in her hip had become unendurable. Her doctor nodded complacently and suggested she was suffering from menopausal complaints. Joyce had always frustrated the family by holding the view that people's physical ailments were either imaginary or exaggerated, and this diagnosis shattered her view of herself. Having despaired over a hysterectomy some years before, she had reached menopause without its obvious sign and had not entirely absorbed its reality. The doctor's denying her pain while confirming her age made her feel out of control. She returned home determined never to complain again. But the intensity of her pain drove her back on her word. This time the doctor asked about her family history. She told him of our mother's recurrent cancers and our father's bursitis. *Bursitis,* the doctor said, and wrote out a prescription to lessen this painful tissue inflammation. The drugs made her groggy without relieving the agony.

As that year moved into the next, the pain tore at her nerve endings. Her power to exist in her habitual ways was radically lessened. She returned to the doctor, who had more x-rays taken. Again he told her that her results had come back with no indication of a problem. He sent her to the hospital for tests. Those results denied her pain as well. To the medical profession, she was indulging her imagination. She needed to find a new hobby, lose a little weight, lighten up.

By this time Joyce leaned on a cane and depended intermittently on a wheelchair. Having raised five children, she had learned to endure. Fortunately, when a knife of pain sliced away the strength she needed to turn the wheel of her car and she flipped over into a ditch, no one else was hurt. Fortunately, too, she hurt herself just enough to be taken by ambulance to a hospital in the adjacent municipality of Langley. After being x-rayed, she met with a new doctor, who diagnosed a neglected kidney cancer that had metastasized to the bone. *Why did you wait so long to seek help?* the doctor asked. *How did you endure the pain?*

I suggested to my lawyer that I would sue her family doctor. The lawyer agreed that this was a reasonable reaction. She also assured me that my chances of doing more than incurring a large debt were slim. The legal tangle would take exhausting years of attempting to penetrate the medical association, long after my sister was gone. Months later, a relative remarked that the doctor, now retired, was actually a nice guy. The Hippocratic oath does not mention *nice*. It focuses on benefiting the patient and bringing relief to those in pain.

From White Rock, my brother-in-law, steady as always, had helped Joyce into their camper van and driven her to the palliative floor of the Vancouver Cancer Clinic. I phoned the hospital from Victoria. *Do you know what palliative means?* the receptionist asked. I thumbed through the dictionary on my desk as she talked. *If your sister would just relax,* the receptionist complained, *she would make it easier on herself.* I thought back on the days when my sister had tried to relax with the diagnosis that she was a middle-aged menopausal neurotic with bursitis. I hoped the receptionist would die slowly and on the street.

From Vancouver, my sister went home to late autumn in White Rock. She seemed vaguely intent on dying in the comfort of her own bedroom. One morning, Bob went to the kitchen to boil water for their breakfast tea. As the phone rang and the kettle boiled, he heard Joyce call his name and the sound of something falling. She was slumped over her walker in the bathroom door. Cancer had chewed its way through the last wedge of hip bone. The ambulance took her to their local hospital, this time to the top floor of Palliative Care.

On that spacious floor, with the sun shining in her shared room, she seemed to regain a degree of contentment. Relieved of the paradoxical responsibility of seeing herself as a burden in the home where she had labored to ease the lives of others, she relaxed into the practical generosities of the nurses and Bob's twice-daily visits. Fed intravenously on the euphoria of morphine, she absorbed the god of dreams. With her pain subdued and her dignity restored, she was expected to live a few weeks. But she clung to life month after month, taking pleasure in the visits of three of her sons and her daughter. I was there to see Joyce's face soften when her son, Doug, brought his two daughters, and when her own daughter, Angela, pulled out a small black kitten she had hidden under her windbreaker.

In the spring of 1990, I traveled frequently across the Strait of Georgia to see my sister. In the comfort of Palliative Care, she was propped up by pillows and medication. During one visit, we laughed easily over photographs of a trip I had made the previous summer to England. Her former caution with its edge of disapproval had vanished. She who had never traveled far from home released herself into vicarious travels. But in the two weeks between this visit and the next, she grew noticeably frailer. No amount of chatter could deny our terror at her body's increasingly rapid journey from robust to sparse, her nervous system's disintegration from lively to vibrating.

Pain takes energy to endure. Its relief brings a new appreciation of the smallest kindness. In Palliative Care, separated from the perpetual motions that turn on a stove or scrape a plate, away from a teen-age daughter who had darkened with her mother's lack of patience, and free of the tension between the maternal dreams for her children and their realities, my sister became emotionally accessible to me for the first time since childhood. We no longer had to work through layers of habit.

I was reminded of a gift Joyce had left on my doorstep shortly before she became noticeably ill and during a dark period in my second divorce. Inside the wrapping was a wooden frame with a picture of a young girl with long brown hair tied back in a white bow. The aproned girl holds up a bowl of grain to six eager geese. Behind them is the prairie that my sister and I had both left behind; above them is a caption: *No act of kindness, however small, is ever wasted.* The girl's sturdy legs and thick brown hair caused me to interpret the gift as a gesture toward my girlhood and my love of birds. But with my own eventual cancer, I came to realize that I had ignored half the message – that Joyce had appreciated my help; when people open up to accept a kindness, their rewards are as plentiful as grains of wheat must seem to hungry geese. The flow of kindness, offering and receiving, creates a river of meaning between two people, symbiotic currents of deep and abiding love.

I couldn't fool myself into thinking that Joyce would rest in the haven of Palliative Care until it was time for her to exchange her slippers for her walking shoes. As cancer gorged itself on her future, I could not bring myself to admit my need to escape, my guilt at having bought a ticket for a two-week holiday in Mexico, and my fear that she would die while I was away. I had trouble meeting her eyes, enlarged orbs that peered knowingly from her skeletal body. She guessed my dilemma and asked me to bring back lots of photographs.

I did not understand cancer that day as well as I would three weeks later. While I was escaping into the dust and heat of Mexico, my sister's flesh was being sucked even closer to the bone. When I returned, her hands had become hauntingly beautiful in their sculptured fluttering. I imagined them whispering over the keys of her grand piano. Her face seemed overwhelmed by her eyes; her lips had thinned to expose her perfect teeth. I carried a chair to her bedside and sat with my face close to hers. She pronounced my name as though it were a tremulous blessing – *Elizabeth.* I felt absolved of sin, the sin of being healthy.

I told her stories about Mexican women, their gentle eyes and open smiles, the way they gather with other women and seem oblivious to their men and endlessly patient with their children. As I spoke, she edged toward me, dragging her life supports an inch at a time, nudging herself toward my thriving flesh. As I touched my palm to her forehead, I noticed that her abundant hair had turned from salt and pepper to sheet-metal gray. Her mouth remained slightly open, her eyes expectant.

I asked if she would like me to take her picture. She nodded with small anxious motions. As the camera clicked her dying into permanence, I shuddered at my audacity. Two years later, when I tidied out a cupboard, the picture I had taken that day caught me off-guard, and other memories of her disappeared in the emotional punch of cancer's final testament. I took the photograph to the fireplace and passed it into the flames. To expiate my guilt, I framed a picture of Joyce that records her final moments in the illusion of health. She looks down on a new granddaughter cradled to her breast, serenity in both their faces.

I wanted to escape from my sister's illness with the same intensity that I wanted to hover over her. The helplessness of watching the sinister progress of disease prompted a sailing trip with friends in the Caribbean. I left for St. Martin before my Mexican tan had faded. In the placid no-land of flight, I realized that my despair, palpable, flew with me. Airlines do not sell insurance for failed happiness.

Once my friends and I had sailed away from the harbor, I ate everything in sight. Food eased the image of Joyce's angular wrists and frightened eyes. With every bite, I encased her and myself in a padded cell of protective flesh. We sailed the warm blue waters together. As the yacht rocked gently in the salty night, I climbed up from the claustrophobic cabin to the deck where I could sleep surrounded by summer air. During the day, I took to swimming long distances, imagining that the enormous turtles beside me had come to give me solace. One day of turquoise water and infinite sand, my friends and I rowed to a tiny island to lunch beneath the thatched roof of a pub. We amused ourselves with a puppy that had ambled away from her siblings. While we ate, three children ran too close to the mother dog, and she left a small laceration on one child's leg. Later, I watched from the water as the pub owner raised his rifle toward the two dogs who had produced the puppies. The male dog had died by the time the crack of the gun reached across the water to my ears. The lactating mother refused to die quickly. She had promises to keep.

I arrived home on a Tuesday and ferried over to the hospital on Wednesday. Joyce's heart still beat but her bones had continued their relentless disintegration. With great effort, she began our final conversation. As if I had been sitting there all the while, she asked, *Where am I going?* Her question implied a loneliness beyond the balm of small escapes and kindling dreams. *You will be wherever Grandma is*, I promised, *and with Mom and Dad too. There's a whole family waiting for you.* I believed what I said so that she would believe it too. My fragile faith in the continuity of the individual spirit surprised me.

Tell people this is scary, she whispered.

To have expected her death would have registered a betrayal of family tradition. *Faith* was the operative word, faith in the ability to struggle on. After all, our maternal grandmother, a prairie pioneer, had lived healthily for ninety-two years before dying in her sleep. Even Mother had managed, against five recurrences of cancer, to achieve her three score and ten. But Joyce, a non-smoker and infrequent drinker, had been the victim of medical incompetence before she became the recipient of its palliative compassion. She clung on until late spring when her fourth and youngest son, Murray, playing in his rock band in Alberta, was tracked down in a basement apartment without a phone. One Thursday this tall, bushy-haired, inarticulate boy surprised her at the foot of the bed, and she responded by regaining all the faculties she had appeared to lose over the months. She called out his name as though he had just returned from an afternoon at college.

The price she had paid to express her joy made itself known when Murray left three days later. On Sunday morning, Bob pushed her down the hall in a wheelchair so that she could look out at the spring flowers. When they returned to her room, she bowed her head and, at age fifty-four, without complaint or good-bye, she stopped breathing.

Joyce did not live to see Angela graduate from college, nor was she there when Bob walked down the aisle arm-in-arm with her. At the altar, he offered his child to a younger man, just as my father had once offered Joyce to him. Ritual and tradition carry new and irrational hope with them. I was surprised to be asked to give the toast at Angela's wedding. It seemed oddly progressive for this family of conservative values to have a woman toast the bride. The invitation opened memories of the years when Joyce, seeking completion, dreamed of mothering a daughter. My toast took the bride back to the days when she had become the beloved prize of my sister. I wanted to give Angela permission to love a mother who had let her down, who had grown disappointed and irritable and then disappeared into hollowed cheeks and shivering bones before her daughter's teen-age eyes.

At Joyce's funeral, I was the only person who wept. Her sons and daughter stood dry-eyed with their father. They shared the expression of people who have experienced an event beyond their comprehension. My tears flowed with the knowledge that my parents' deaths had brought me. I would never again hear my sister's voice or see her face change expression when I entered her room. She was the first in our family to be cremated. Where would she find the amazing grace the soloist had promised? When the pallbearers lowered the coffin lid to cover her frail remains, I followed her down the church aisle alone and watched the hearse disappear into the late spring sunshine. Her ashes mingle now with the Pacific Ocean, off the coast of Oregon, a place where she and Bob shared special times. There is no gravestone for ritual visits and the laying of flowers. On the ferry home after the funeral, I watched from the deck as the earth turned away from the light, making room for someone else's dawning.

We three sisters had gathered only twice before when Joyce was central to the occasion. I had invited Lynne to visit the hospital with me as a gift to Joyce of solidarity. The other gathering had been many years earlier, when Lynne and I stood together in our new dresses while Joyce and Bob exchanged the words that would alter their lives. After the groom kissed the bride, Joyce went into the church vestibule to change into her going-away suit. She was going away from her parents' family to her own, trading a life of being done to for a life of doing for, beginning her servitude younger than most.

All her life, Joyce had an extraordinary degree of modesty. During her marriage, she remained riveted to the idea of proving her virtue. No one to my knowledge ever saw her nude, except perhaps her husband, the doctors, and, on two occasions, myself. This seems odd to me now, since she and I slept for four years in a bed that sagged toward the center and caused no end of riled sensitivities.

The first time I saw her nude was on that wedding day, when she stepped out of her layers of white lace and into her blue going-away suit. I realized to my relief that she too had pubic hair. Having barely entered teenhood, I felt charged with gratitude that this sister of mine, this beautiful bride, this gruff and reluctant high school dropout, had the same body as I had been surprised to discover on myself. My relief that I was normal and that she was loved was too much, and I collapsed in tears. *What are you bawling about?* she asked in a voice tinged with disgust. *I'm going to miss you,* I told her as my nose dripped onto my new dress. *I doubt it,* she replied, and huffed off to begin her new life.

Decades later, in Palliative Care, I attempted to leave her room for a brief walk in the sunshine. *Don't go,* she said in a small voice. *I'll be back soon,* I assured her. *Don't go,* she repeated. Her request erased the shame of nights long ago when my sleep-heavy body had rolled toward hers in the sagging bed and she had let loose her frustration as I crossed the invisible line into a war zone.

I saw her nude again when the serenity of morphine had taken her back to childhood. I entered her room one afternoon to discover her talking to herself in the voice of a child. She had drawn her hospital gown up to eye level and was attempting to arrange what she thought was a carefully pleated skirt. The blankets lay tangled about her feet. Her face softened when she saw me, and she returned to semi-adulthood, but not to an awareness of her body. I knew her embarrassment would know no bounds, if her embarrassed self could still be found, and I stooped to sweep the covers over her nakedness. The image of her mount of Venus stayed with me, rich as the prairie soil we were born to, hiding the passage that had birthed five children, the births that denied her extinction.

I realize that Joyce is responsible in part for my reaction to the world. I did not always agree with her and often I felt wounded by her conservative and judgmental outlook, but in some formerly unexamined corner of my heart, I have always loved her. We are inextricably bound by our childhood experience. She was not erased for me by her death, but remains an inescapable part of my being. The end of her life brought us home to the secret essence of our beginnings.

Sisters become the eyes of time. Returning home to each other, we converge to prove that the way is long but the time is short. Memories spill into my tomorrows as I travel with Joyce now. She makes me valuable.

❧ 4 ❧

Sweet Bird of Health

In the summer of 1986 I rented a rusty bicycle in Bali to visit the Valley of White Cranes. I pedaled into the late afternoon over a bumpy road where I caught unforgettable glimpses of Balinese people. A small man who walked like a dancer kept his flock of geese marching alongside the treacherous roadway by carrying a long stick with a white flag on it. He never struck his eager flock; he kept it in line by waving the flag within their vision. Not one goose lost its life to the two-way traffic that crammed into one lane. I figured if a gaggle of geese could travel unscathed to its destination, so could I. But as the light and traffic dimmed, my determination began to fade. I feared I would not find the famous birds before they nested down for the night that falls so suddenly near the equator.

My spirits were rejuvenated by the sight of an elderly, bare-breasted Balinese woman who leaned her fragile body into the spray from a small waterfall. As I watched her enjoy her evening shower, I felt a renewed sense of pleasure in my journey. I was reminded at the age of forty-five how beautiful old age can be. Swerving and bouncing between potholes, I saw just ahead of me an old Balinese man who seemed to be entranced by something I could not see. I climbed off my bicycle to ask him directions to the

Valley of White Cranes, flapping my arms like a bird to convey my meaning. He gestured toward the sky. Above me I saw a cornucopia of bird life, white feathers mingled with the treescape. The cranes had been hovering all the while.

One may be on the lookout for a malignancy, but its being there is nevertheless overwhelming. *Overwhelm* was the word my acupuncturist used to tell me I was in shock. It was December of 1995, and I had recently been biopsed and diagnosed with a lung cancer near my mediastinum, the space between my ribs, smack dab in the center of pulsating things.

Sorrow was the first feeling I acknowledged after the shock subsided. How would Noel manage without me? How could I tell my old Airedale, Chance, that she would probably outlive me? How could I bear to have someone else drive off in my car, open my office door, come home to our house? A need for the milk of human kindness caused me to see with new eyes. On the instant, friends and ex-lovers were forgiven their trespasses. Tugboats called out to me with childish hope as they worked their way up the Strait of Juan de Fuca during my morning walk: *I think I can, I think I can.*

Shame, oddly enough, replaced my sorrow. In the 1990s women were not supposed to allow themselves to be victims of anything. I had done too much. I had done too little. I had wavered. I was a non-smoking, health-food eating, sports-oriented woman with a fulfilling relationship and a stimulating career. No one smoked around me anymore, and radon gas was non-existent in my corner of the world. I downed my vitamins with breakfast and I breathed the cleanest air on the planet. I had secretly puffed a few cigarettes in the aftermath of divorce and had even toked on happy herbs (as my respirologist called them) during my years in

Cambridge in the late 1960s. I had also spent the odd night as a couch potato, eating banana and peanut-butter sandwiches in front of the television. But what had I done to deserve the death penalty? As I contemplated the nature of justice, time grew thick and still. My toenails began to peer over the tops of my toes when I forgot to cut them. I stared at them, as though they belonged to someone else.

Then anger erupted, mingled with self-pity, as word of my illness traveled the grapevine of friends and colleagues. In my imagination everyone else was simply curious, engulfed in the busyness of life, oblivious to my despair. I wanted to be normal, over *there* instead of over *here*. I saved a special fury for those who phoned to ask, *Soooo, how are you?* What was I to say? Between answering calls, I wrote a note to my doctor, telling her I would be seeking help from a new general practitioner. After all, she had refused me an x-ray during the spring and summer and early fall of 1994, telling me my cough was just an allergy. In November, my x-ray showed a serious pneumonia, a diagnosis that left me relieved to have had my cough acknowledged. But then, as December unfolded, she told me that cancer was a distinct possibility. She had thought me too young and too fit to have this particular cancer. But I too was responsible. In war with a haunting terror in my gut, I had rationalized that my cough would disappear.

No, I couldn't possibly be sick. Noel had moved recently from Vancouver so that we could be together, a couple, after three years of sharing weekend commutes. We did all the things couples do: renovating a house, buying a van, getting season's tickets to the opera, and pledging our eternal love. Besides, I had just acquired a sizable grant and had begun work on my Ph.D. Noel had landed a challenging job. We were set. I clung to the notion that constructive people do not get cancer. When nothing could arrest my cough –

not rest, not exercise, not medication, not even love — I was reminded of a conversation I'd had with Lynne some years before. We had shared fantasies about who we would like to be if we were not ourselves. She said she wanted to be Whitney Houston and I said I wanted to be Barbara Frum. Frum's own cancer didn't reach public knowledge until a decade later.

Disillusioned, I was forced to accept that happiness and health are not interconnected in the simple ways I had imagined. Happy thoughts may help recovery but they are not enough. Genetics, environment, and the vast unknown pack a mighty wallop too. I began to move through the days in slow motion, a one-way mirror between myself and others. Concentration was a thing of the past, thoughts were hard to separate, the right words difficult to find. My eyes glazed over when I tried to follow a movie or read a book.

The phone startled me from this freeze-dried state. A bed was waiting in the only available space in the hospital, the geriatric ward. I arranged a squash game, played with intensity, drove to the hospital, and climbed into bed among the elderly. Next to me was a grandmotherly woman who spoke lovingly with the white-haired man who visited her. I caught bits of their conversation and marveled at their playful camaraderie. She told me later that they were newlyweds who had discovered each other after their former mates had died and all their children had left home. She suggested with a shy smile that my man adored me. She filled me with a longing for my tomorrows.

Next morning on the operating-room table, the respirologist took a biopsy that confirmed what the radiologist had suspected — a slow-growing cancer in a dangerous location. The following day, a scan showed the cancer was extensive but contained. After being put on the long list of people who wait to pass through the doors of the cancer clinic, I packed my bag and went up to Whistler Mountain to ski my way to health in the fresh air. Instead I again came down with raging pneumonia and became one of the few sober people (besides the medical staff) in Emergency at Vancouver General Hospital on New Year's Eve. The respirologist there called me when I returned to Victoria to inquire after my health. With his call, my faith in the compassion of the medical profession began, with reservation, to be restored.

The radiation oncologist at the cancer clinic suggested that I see yet another specialist in the round of medical musical chairs, a surgeon. If the removal of my right lung was possible, this would raise my 15 percent chance of survival to 40 percent. Early in 1995, I was put on an emergency list, sent home, and left to idle away day after dreary day until January turned into February. I swung between wanting the surgery immediately, before I metastasized, and wanting to hold onto my newly appreciated lung. Nor had I appreciated my unscarred chest until a friend asked about the blade that would separate my two halves. I thought of my mother chopping up chicken breasts for dinner.

In early February the surgeon did exploratory surgery – a horizontal slice at the base of my neck, the beginnings of decapitation. When I awoke, the anesthesiologist grinned down on me. *It looks good*, he said. *Lymph nodes are clean.* The surgeon warned me that removing a lobe would be high-risk surgery. I imagined his nicking my heart, blood soaking the operating table. In my mind's eye, I watched the knife accidentally puncture my lung. It deflated like a ruined soufflé while I gasped for air. All this for less than a 50 percent chance at life. I feigned appreciation and tried to ignore the operation date. At least February thirteenth wasn't a Friday, I consoled myself.

Along with my man and my toothbrush, I took into hospital two gifts and the knowledge that cancer cannot be divided. *All* the tumor and its immediate periphery would be removed or nothing. One friend, Jenny, gave me a talisman she had been given by the Bedouin when, as a young woman in her twenties, she crossed the North African desert. Another friend, Trudy, gave me a diamond ring her grandmother had worn to safety when, in France, she lived through two world wars. With these symbols of strength and endurance, I submitted once again to shutting down the pain center in my brain. As I lay inert, the surgeon sawed through my bodice, neck to navel. Cleavage took on new meaning.

Having pried open my ribs, the doctor discovered what the x-ray had not revealed – a tentacle of cancer had wrapped its sinister arm around my heart. This flirtation of sorts had erupted during the nine months since I had begun to frequent my general practitioner's office with a cough. Cancer had wrapped itself around my ascending aorta and my superior vena cava, parts of my female heart. The tumor was inoperable. I was stapled, stitched, and returned to my room.

When my eyelids overcame the anesthetic, I looked into the sorrowful blue of Noel's eyes. His imagination struck out against the current of our despair: *Now when you recover you'll have two lungs instead of one.* We never spoke the word *inoperable.* We never planned for death. He simply exuded in silence a depth of caring that surpasses words. I pressed the portable morphine button that made breathing bearable, relief at six-second intervals.

Every day brought a new country of discomfort and fear. On Tuesday I allowed a limited reality to roam about my psyche, one that excluded thoughts of a terminal diagnosis. Instead I focused my disappointment on the immediate and called for a bed pan. The nurse suggested that I use the commode chair because I might dribble on the sheets. Pride made me stupid. I shuffled to the bathroom. Without morphine, I carried a concrete block of pain. Faced with the familiar sight of the toilet, I learned about the number of muscles required to bend the knees ever so slightly and to breathe all the while – in and out, in and out – moving severed flesh, nerves, and bone.

On Wednesday the limits of my reality expanded; all the nerve endings in my brain exploded against my misfortune. I asked for my migraine medication. Six nurses in succession had not heard of it. They decided unanimously that it did not exist. The overworked nurse of the moment shot me with Gravol. As I waited for visitors, not knowing about the Do Not Disturb sign taped to my closed door, the Gravol took effect. In late afternoon, a new nurse arrived and with her my familiar pink migraine pills. *I too suffer migraines,* she said cheerfully.

Rejuvenated, I entertained myself by calling my own voice mail at the college. There was one message only. A voice programmed to cover my department announced that unfortunately my cancer had spread, making my tumor inoperable, and that people should visit soon if they planned to visit at all. As my saliva evaporated, I sunk back in stupor. But on Thursday when my colleagues arrived with flowers, fruit, and stories, they brought the relief of forgetfulness. This family of sorts buoyed me with their healing strength and energizing chatter.

Every day during these emotional ups and downs, one of my four doctors dropped by my room. My surgeon, for example, came to express his regret that the tumor's spread had not been accurately calculated. He explained that the limitations of x-ray made diagnosis difficult. He encouraged me to brave the simultaneous chemotherapy and radiation treatments by two oncologists, a tag team. My general practitioner, rather than escape a confrontation with me, came through a snowstorm to distract me with stories of a marvelous birthing she had attended and a remarkable breast reconstruction after a mastectomy. My respirologist came by daily, and we talked of the book we had both recently read. He brought as well suggestions of hope, assuring me that he had seen worse than me recover. He had known one woman, older and less healthy than I was, to last nine years. The anesthesiologist relaxed in a chair, telling me bedtime stories of medical oddities – a brain surgeon, for example, who himself had got brain cancer and kept his tumor on his desk to express the recuperative power of surgery to frightened patients. Together these doctors let me know they were doing what they could to find a pathway for my recovery.

Between visitors, Noel wheeled me down to the cancer clinic where I was to begin treatments toward a remission – a trial test of simultaneous high-dosage chemotherapy and radiation. The chemotherapy oncologist had to turn me away, however; I was too recently cut open to risk the violent vomiting that usually accompanies toxic injections in heavy dosages. Once again I was ambivalent. I wanted to risk everything to avoid the spread of malignant cells; I wanted to go home and hide. I wanted everything to be as it was before. I was given a two-week reprieve.

Noel decided on Friday that my chances of recovery, after five days in hospital, would be enhanced if I were at home in our airy new bedroom with its windows that look out on cedar trees and visiting birds. When no one would discharge me, he *borrowed* a wheelchair from the hall and bundled me in my favorite quilt. Propped up like the egg of an endangered species, I felt a surge of security sitting next to him in our van until we began to move forward. My chest seemed to open with each infinitesimal bump, threatening to spill my heart into my lap. As we crawled into the driveway, raindrops spattered the windshield, another Victoria springtime in the midst of a Canadian winter. We tucked a pillow against my chest, collected Chance, and walked the long, long distance of two house lengths to Beacon Hill Park. As I shuffled along, clutching my pillow, terrified to sneeze or turn my head, an eleven-year-old neighbor called out, *Look Mommy, Elizabeth's had a baby!* The mother told me later that she had been certain I had lost a breast to cancer. So far I had lost nothing except the illusion of a certain future.

In exchange for this loss, I received two unexpected gifts that night as I lay immobile on the couch. A lengthy fax arrived from a friend in Saudi Arabia. She took me on vicarious travels through a culture alien to my own. I wept as I watched her children light candles and pray for my survival; I followed her into the sea and fell asleep exploring exotic fish; I battled alongside her against a bureaucracy that denied the rights of women. The second gift was the arrival of a friend from Vancouver. She had lugged considerable food from her car to our refrigerator before she began to cook. After she had served us a magnificent meal, filled the freezer, and cleaned the kitchen, she stole away into the dawn. These are but two of many friends who taught me about the precious role of caregiver. Many people need only know that their help is welcome to open the floodgates of their healing powers. They made my operation less painful and my anticipation of therapy less terrifying. They made me feel worth saving.

Chemotherapy is a nightmare that parallels the birthing process: one must go through a brief hell for the joy of reaching an important goal. Like all unspeakable twists of fate, it is somehow endurable. I was part of a trial that had begun eight months before, combining chemotherapy and radiation therapy for non-small-cell lung cancer. As radiation breaks down the tumor so it can be flushed from the body, chemotherapy attacks the invisible microbes that move through the system to lodge in other organs. People seldom die from a localized lung tumor. The menace comes from metastases, when stray cancer cells break off and tumble into such organs as the liver or the brain, organs that have no duplicates. Metastasis is the Nazi of the cancer world; hungry for power, these uncharitable cells scour the body for vulnerable places to invade.

One must acquire a faith in tomorrow to survive a clinical trial emotionally. Because it is a trial, little statistical clarity exists. A computer scientist once suggested, however, that to take statistics seriously one must accept the idea that every individual has one testicle and one breast. Without faith in the trial's success, how could I offer up my veins to welcome for a second, third, fourth, and fifth time the poisoned needle? How could I spend the week taking anti-nausea pills, and moving a bit of food from platter to quivering palate? Nausea followed me all the days of my new life.

The side effects of chemotherapies differ with each cancer. Mine included serious dehydration, possible deafness, heart damage, loss of feeling in fingers and toes, kidney and liver damage, and other no less daunting afflictions. I put one foot in front of the other and walked along the water's edge in rhythm with my arthritic dog. I was blessed in that I did not suffer beyond my ability to ready my body for the following week's dosage. And I was doubly blessed by the company of Noel, who arranged time away from his new job to support me each Tuesday morning when I had the injection. He took notes as I spoke with the doctors, asked for answers that I would need to survive the week, and remembered crucial facts when my eyes glazed over. How could I teach if I became deaf? How could I grade papers with numb hands? We labored to balance the negative possibilities against the odds of prolonged survival.

The chemotherapy room has a circle of adjustable recliner chairs, padded to comfort the patient who must sit for up to three hours being hydrated and poisoned by a needle that bites into the bony back of the hand. Left hand this week, right hand next. One patient in the circle munched on candies as he propped up his severely swollen ankles; another tossed off her scarf to share her newly exposed scalp and the stray hairs that still protruded from it; another joked away her hysteria with her husband; another sat stern and silent in her tailored smile; yet another talked of his coming trip to England.

During my second chemotherapy treatment, I confided in my oncologist, Heidi, that my sweetie's fiftieth birthday was a week away and I was sorry I would be unable to enjoy the party I had arranged from bed. Each friend was bringing food and a glass, and I was providing wine and coffee. The invitations and arrangements had been organized on a cordless phone during my hours in bed. Heidi swung into action to make sure I would be well enough to be up and about during what was usually my most inactive time – the hours between dinner and sleep. She organized my treatments and hydration so that I could share the celebration. Noel had no idea about the wine hidden in the basement or the paper plates, napkins, and birthday candles stuffed in the back of a closet. By five o'clock on the day of the party, I felt frail but smug. While I meditated for twenty minutes, I could not push away the thought that I had forgotten to order the second most important ingredient, after friends, for a birthday party. The local bakery seemed delighted to hear from a desperate shopper just before closing time. They happened to have a beautiful carrot cake to feed forty guests, decorated for a birthday but baked for the wrong Saturday. I could send a friend to pick it up. Noel happily overlooked the one small glitch: it had blue and red plaid icing.

Nurses who administer chemotherapy have the daunting task of making patients relax. They are masters of diplomacy, quick to bring a heating pad to cover hand and needle, to offer sedatives to those nauseated with fear, and to bring food to those with an appetite. I spent my time reading short stories and convincing myself that I looked forward to lunch. Eating is a constant challenge for patients as their scales dip and their bodies wither with an acute sensitivity to the smells of food. I almost swooned at the odor of basmati rice, a food I had never before been conscious of smelling. But I could indulge with abandon in extravagant ice creams. Peanut-butter and banana sandwiches were no longer the enemy. Unfortunately my fantasy foods often seemed better in the abstract. When I did not lose my hair or need hospitalization, I worried that the chemotherapy was not working. Heidi assured me that these side effects are not a measure of how well the chemotherapy is blasting away the cancer cells, distinguishing them from the healthy cells that grow at a slower rate.

The radiation laboratory was less personal and more awesome than the chemotherapy room. Patients sat in a waiting room in the company of family, friends, and magazines, listening for their names to be called. One woman coughed with a deep and hollow bark that made the loose skin quiver on her wasted arms. Two other women, who often accompanied each other, wore colorful baseball caps to cover their baldness and ample make-up to camouflage the damage that chemotherapy and radiation therapy do to the skin. To give themselves attitude, they wore outrageous earrings. They reminded me of a garden I had once seen blossoming under the fluorescent lights in the depths of a Cape Breton coal mine, planted by an old-timer who recognized in all that darkness a need for beauty.

Coughing, skin rashes, fatigue, and nausea are common signs of radiation sickness. Apart from bone-weary exhaustion, however, I suffered only a mild throat irritation, rather like the teary lump that accompanies a sad movie. I was considered fortunate. My grandmother used to tell me not to leave the house unless I was wearing clean underpants; I might be involved in a car accident and the medical staff would question my mother's parenting skills. If I were to have grandchildren, I would tell them not to leave the house without being physically fit in case they might be involved in an energy-sapping disease. When the quantity of life is threatened, the quality becomes crucial to motivation and stamina. Just as my grandmother was concerned with the laundry and our family pride, so I became concerned with my immunity and my body's recuperative powers.

On my initial visit for radiation therapy, I was tattooed. Not a bird, not a plane, but superdot, a freckle of indelible ink, marked the heart of my tumor. A laboratory technician made me a partial body mold that would encase my back to keep me still while I was being subjected to the powerful rays, since any movement could cause the radiation to miss its precious mark and kill healthy cells. I stretched out on a plastic sheet while the technician sprayed a foam between the plastic and the stretcher. In seconds, the dampness expanded and solidified to form a comfortable likeness of my back. A section of the mold was then carved out to allow the radiation to penetrate the tumor while still protecting as much healthy tissue as possible.

Snug in my mold, alone in the spacious room that houses the radiation equipment, I listened to the click of machinery moving around me and the buzzer that signaled the penetration of invisible rays. The process was lonely and vaguely unreal. I felt as though I were playing at being sick, taking part in a postmodern drama. I was actually being given a curative dose, the maximum localized radiation that human flesh can withstand. No room for error here.

Once my twenty days of radiation therapy ended, both oncologists examined my new x-ray. *This is as good as it gets*, said Stefan, the radiation oncologist. I hoped he meant that my response equaled his highest expectation, not that I was doing poorly and would do no better. I could not brave the question that would have clarified the point, but I was comforted by his confident look. Heidi decided chemotherapy treatments were negotiable now that my tumor had shrunk from sight. I could quit, she explained. Further chemotherapy would risk permanent damage to my still healthy organs and nerve tissues, but it could also protect me against metastases. She assured me I had absorbed a considerable dosage of chemotherapy already. I alone had to make the choice, knowing that one remaining malignant cell could begin the ordeal all over again. If my cancer returned soon, it would be with a vengeance that resulted from the few Herculean cells that managed to survive the chemotherapy. With considerable apprehension, I chose to walk away.

My treatments ended with the month of April 1995. Since then I have had to adapt to being easily tired, slightly breathless, and often frightened. These are not traits I admire. I live now with the possibility of the tumor's return and the reality that I have used up my allotment of radiation on the primary site. I eventually sought out alternative therapies to complement the mainstream medical practices. The healing powers of acupuncture, massage, naturopathy, and yoga suggest that the mind plays a role in health that matches the power of the body. Science and healing became Siamese twins in my progress toward remission.

My acupuncturist, Elena, a former pediatric nurse for leukemia patients, has an encyclopedic knowledge of both conventional and alternative treatments. With her intuitive sense of physical and spiritual well-being, she tells me to live each day with full respect for its importance. This task is more daunting than one might imagine. My massage therapists, Catherine and Jan, knead me into a willing calm that enables me to begin afresh each week. My naturopathic physician, Bruce, gives me diluted substances to steady my organs. My yoga teacher, Marie, shows me how to stretch my limbs, massage my organs, and breathe in health and tranquillity. All the while my new general practitioner, Bill, keeps watch.

Some days, however, I slip into despondency. I awaken with dread that yesterday's cough might be today's pneumonia, that a migraine might hint at brain metastasis, that the flush of fear I felt before my initial diagnosis might return to remind me that the body knows beforehand what the mind has to be told. I try to be confident about my future in the hope that we do in fact become the person we aspire to be. As I speed up my morning walk, I adapt to shortened breathing patterns – premonitions of suffocation. In June 1995, I traveled to Massachusetts to check out recent publications on treatments and statistics for my particular cancer and was discouraged yet again by the lack of improvement in survival rates. In July 1995, I sailed off Cortes Island with Noel and felt omnipotent in the pristine waters of Desolation Sound. One year later, I have joined the Y to limber my reflexes, expand my lung power, and build strength. I continue to make the bed, wash the clothes, and shop for groceries.

But I reside now in a stranger's body. We are only beginning to know each other. I have a lung that betrayed me, even perhaps as I betrayed it. I wear a scar that penetrates my courage as well as my breast. I am the same and yet forever changed. But steadily melting away these moments of fear is a growing trickle of inexplicable hope. Sweet bird of health, be with me.

5

The Perfection
of Hope

S cientists are doubters. With skepticism they labor to substantiate facts that eventually create statistics, forecasting, for example, the cause, process, and prognosis of a disease. Statistics, by their nature, offer information on the generic experience but not on personal idiosyncrasies. Medical scientists question the obvious, re-examine the data, and duplicate results in double-blind studies. They acquire scientific proof through precisely controlled repetitions. Cancer patients depend on this discipline for diagnoses and treatments. But the uniqueness of the singular patient is lost in the numbers game, and with it the optimism necessary for day-to-day survival.

The variations that make one person irrevocably different from another came home to me when my respirologist, Bruce Sanders, asked me in the hospital emergency room if I smoked. *Well not really*, I told him. *I've had a cigarette at a party or when I was stressed out about my personal life. But not for years.* He interrupted me to define a smoker as someone who smokes a pack a day over a period of years. *Oh!* I said, relieved, wondering if this meant that I could go home rather than into the bowels of the hospital for further tests. *I've never smoked a whole package in a day*, I said, elated. *I've hardly ever bought a package. I mostly bummed one or two. A cigarette, not a package.* Behind my nervous chatter, I was silently begging the doctor to recant his opinion that I might have lung cancer.

It could be tuberculosis, he said, relieving my terror in spite of the moans that came from the next cubicle. *I had a student whose nose bled all over her exam,* I told him. *She lives on the Saanich reserve and had been diagnosed with TB and didn't want to lose her semester by missing her final, and I helped her from the classroom,* I babbled. *We'll do tests,* the doctor said. After he pulled the curtain aside, he turned back for a moment: *These new strains of TB can be worse than cancer, harder to eradicate.*

Although Dr. Sanders eventually defined me as someone who had not been much of a smoker, I felt defensive, duplicitous, and guilty. I thought about second-hand smoke and the academic offices where I had worked to help my first husband through school. I had sat amid a crowd of zoologists, botanists, and microbiologists. Often they puffed cigarettes while I banged on the typewriter. They read their articles over my shoulder as I typed them. When I got home, I sat with my husband as he worked toward his architectural degree at his drafting table, cigarette between his lips, while I read the novels and short stories assigned for his literature class. I felt tricked to have contracted the very thing heavy smokers dread – inoperable lung cancer. *Inoperable* is not a synonym for death, but it's a warning that remission rather than cure may be the outcome of medical help, and that the search for extended life would require my own vigilance after the treatments were finished.

Simultaneous chemotherapy and radiation treatment was offered to me because I was fit in other ways. Although it seems ironic to be considered healthy enough for cancer treatments, this is an important point. If the liver and kidneys are healthy to start with, for example, the body stands a better chance of supporting recovery or remission of other organs. All those hours running around a squash or tennis court and skiing and walking my dog had not been wasted. Fitness got me through the clinic treatments and out the door without a stretcher or a wheelchair. I then lay down on the tables of alternative therapists.

The process of destroying cancer had put considerable stress on my nerves, especially on my sense of control over my own body. Alternative therapies offer holistic healing, connecting mind, body, and spirit. These complementary treatments help restore a sense of well-being. Friends gave me the names of various therapists; one therapist referred me to another; soon I had a full schedule of support. My incentive came from a small voice of hope that gained volume and clarity with each infinitesimal change for the better. As anyone recovering from surgery, chemotherapy, and radiation knows, forward motion gains momentum in the sanctuary of hope.

Hope is the stuff on which productive energy is built. The confidence it engenders allows a patient to separate rewarding activities from social pressures, to know when to push and when to fall back, to favor process over a momentary end. Denial, on the other hand, creates frenetic movement or total apathy. It may masquerade as acceptance, but anger and fear hover beneath denial, poisoning the fragile soil in which optimism roots itself.

My goal has been to polish a frame of mind that imagines cancer as a bathtub ring – a result of pollutants, something that can be made to disappear with the right cleansers, a little discipline, and a realistic awareness that it takes repeated effort to keep clean. The initial cleansing came from conventional treatments that killed off the toxic cells but left a residue of their own. The complementary processes helped me return to a comfortable life. Instead of wondering why I had bothered to avoid fatty foods, spend restorative time in the Land of Nod, and exercise daily, I reminded myself that these activities had facilitated my recovery. Having walked in the hobbled boots of the misdiagnosed, I learned that a patient, however exhausted and dependent, can cushion her journey to recovery by seeking the help of qualified healers who alter the patient's point of view as well as her balance of energies. Truth in uniqueness, in instinctual awareness, is what complementary therapists strive to discover and sustain. As k.d. lang says, *There's no place to find truth, except in your soul and your instincts.*

I discovered that the courage to ignore social assumptions and to maintain my sense of uniqueness wore thin at times, especially in confrontation with grim statistics. I had to separate myself emotionally from newspaper stories that told me lung cancer was on the rise among women and ranked as a major cause of death, up there with heart disease and breast cancer. The news never seemed to share the reality that lung cancer also afflicts women who have never smoked, as two of my acquaintances proved. Or that patients who smoked heavily may be cured completely, as two other acquaintances demonstrated.

One of these women had a relatively simple surgery after she had quit smoking. Minus one lobe, she returned to her former life with less breath and a sore chest, but has suffered no further setbacks. Another woman smoked two packs a day for thirty years before her cancer was diagnosed. It simply disappeared. She told me she accomplished this without medical help, but with two changes. She quit her job as a flight attendant, a job in which she had been immersed in second-hand smoke as well as her own before smoking was prohibited on flights, and she began walking two miles a day. Her doctors were baffled and remained silent about this apparent miracle, perhaps to discourage smokers from feeling confident.

In spite of the power of statistics, I find that one or two success stories, especially with lung cancer, strengthen my resolve to live a healthy life no matter how my history differs from those who have recovered. I keep in mind my chemotherapist's story about the woman who finally had to be told to go away after surviving inoperable lung cancer for twenty-nine years. Smoking assists many cancers and inhibits many cures (even complicating recovery from surgery), but women should not be lulled, as I was, by their non-smoker status or their general fitness into ignoring bodily changes that persist – even when a doctor offers vague reassurance.

In the wake of my surgery, morphine became my life line. After two weeks on the drug, I began to have fleeting visions of rats jumping from corners of the bedroom, disappearing midair. I dreamed that I cycled down a dark country road. Behind me I recognized the sound of a wheelchair being propelled at great speed by stronger arms than my own. I could barely glimpse my competitor on a night road made darker by a curtain of trees. As the menace overtook me, I suffocated in its power. When I awoke in darkness, I recognized my fear of being permanently disabled by cancer.

It was sometime after this dream, and before I had completed my treatments in the cancer clinic, that I began to look into alternative therapies. I had come to understand that, having been treated with whatever oncologists decide is appropriate to a particular cancer, a patient is left to face alone the physical and emotional aftermath.

Complementary therapies fortified me against the conventional treatment's abuse of my healthy organs. I learned to absorb healing energies and sustain precious hope. Alternative therapists focus on the individual as a whole and not on the cancerous organ as a singular enemy, freeing the patient to be a statistical exception. Conjuring up my own path to wellness began to strengthen my immune system (the main prevention against all illness) and to regain the necessary belief that recovery, at least to some extent, was within my control. Northrop Frye suggested that *all hope is based on fiction. It has no facts to go on. It is where the creative impulse takes over.* With lung cancer, medical science suggests I have an 80 percent chance of dying: Beware! Alternative therapy suggests I have a 20 percent chance of cure. Go for it!

An essential companion is someone to link traditional and complementary treatments into one effective process. In my case, a general practitioner, Bill Cavers, proved himself a Renaissance man of health care. He expressed a belief in the methods of science and the complicit powers of the spirit. Inquisitive and approachable, he welcomed my questions and opinions and used humor to soften his explanation of my difficult prognosis (such as the reality that metastasis is a threat that may lessen with time but never disappears). He shared his knowledge of my cancer, listened to my program of healing, and suggested I consider observation and balance as the operative goals – monitor today and believe in tomorrow. He is the funnel through which traditional and nontraditional treatments find a meeting place, the trusted gatekeeper of my future health.

Between visits to medical scientists and alternative therapists, I actively contributed to my own health. Exercise keeps the blood moving, the organs massaged, and the flesh solid as it elevates the spirit. The literature suggests that cancer patients should exercise to the point of sweating but not to the point of dizziness – a warning of dehydration or oxygen deprivation. Copious amounts of purified water protect me from dehydration.

Shortly after dawn each day I meander by the water's edge along the Strait of Juan de Fuca, meditating and visualizing. In the evening, as the sun dips into the horizon, I walk with friends – needing company, wanting conversation, moving as fast as I can. Once my heart has slowed and my body cooled, I can eat a whale and sleep a season. These simple comforts may not guarantee me a centenarian's stretch, but they relieve physical discomfort and emotional pain by expanding the potential for fulfillment.

My mantra for meditation came serendipitously one day on my way to the chemotherapy room. On the car radio I heard a writer advise, *Go slowly and all good things will come to you.* Although I never learned the writer's name, the words struck home, and I have acquired the habit of repeating them whenever I find myself caught up in congested traffic or grocery lineups. The effect is instant: a casting away of ticking time, a calm involvement in the now, a recognition of the inevitable foibles of human interaction.

Before I received my first post-treatment x-ray, which revealed my apparently tumor-free lung, I learned with practice to visualize. I needed a vision that did not involve the battle raging between good and bad cells frequently found on healing tapes and in books on visualization. I wanted to support my medical treatments; images of war destroyed this sense of involvement. My vision was of a large iceberg (tumor) on which the sun shone (radiation therapy) and around which the waves (healthy cells) lapped to erode its edges. Small boats (lymph nodes) fought against being sucked into the overwhelming force of the iceberg's journey (metastases). All the while a warm and powerful wind (chemotherapy) swirled around the iceberg, disrupting the stability of everything in its path while shrinking the icy cathedral. I could turn up the sunbeams or turn down the wind with my imagination. I became the goddess of my own destiny. Even now the sight of placid waters under a gentle sun eases my chest muscles. Obviously each patient and each cancer needs an individual vision.

My first major foray into Eastern philosophy began at the suggestion of a colleague, Kathleen Ryan, diagnosed with inoperable lung cancer a year before my own diagnosis. She sent me to her acupuncturist, Elena. The philosophy of acupuncture involves inquiring about the patient's emotional response to her world. In essence, the therapist begins with a knowledge of the patient's sense of her own being before taking her pulses and treating her for the blocks that stem the flow of her energy. Although I had spent too many years in the academic world to give myself over quickly to the concept of an energy field I could not see, Elena's intelligence and wisdom soon won my confidence. I remembered my colleague telling me that she confided to Elena things she had never told anyone. I could not imagine myself telling a stranger my secrets, but with the loneliness of cancer and the trust that Elena engendered, I found myself owning up to secret fears and dreams. I told her I often felt I had been cured but was afraid to say so because I would look foolish if the cancer recurred or spread. She smiled wryly and agreed it would be terrible to have spent my remaining months or years in happy contentment.

Many of my friends, with problems ranging from rheumatoid arthritis to depression, have begun visiting Elena to escape my long-winded praise. She treats each of us differently, having no pat answers and an ability to hear each individual cry. She suggested that I open up to love. This struck me as odd advice to offer a woman who was in a meaningful relationship with a man who had moved from his city to hers so they could be together. As my treatments continued at the clinic, Elena coaxed me into seeing that I would have to depend on others for a while, strangers and friends alike. She taught me to use my instincts in trusting people's concern, in knowing when to leave the key under the mat. I feared that openness might lead to unwanted opinions and gossip; I discovered the more I opened the door on my privacy, the more the doors of trust opened for me.

Acupuncture relies on the presence of endorphins, the body's natural antidote to pain. A tiny needle taps into the blocked meridian, just below the skin's surface, releasing endorphins, relaxing the pain centers of the body, and bringing serenity to the patient's nervous system. One patient finds herself energized to accomplish tasks she couldn't face; another feels a deep need to catch up on rest. If certain needle points cause discomfort, Elena finds another route to unblocking a particular meridian. We had to agree to disagree on the importance of reaching a vital energy center through my toes; I am a person in perpetual lust for a foot massage, and I could not bear the idea of someone putting needles in my toes. Taking one hand at a time, Elena listens to my eight pulses with the attention of a sheep dog on its herd. With acupressure she can melt away a migraine and make me wonder at a medical system that provides pills for the asking but does little to fund the invaluable services of a trained acupuncturist.

When I am frail, Elena uses moxibustion (or moxa), a gentle process often used on children and the seriously ill. Moxa is a herb that looks like a pinch of dried brown tobacco. Lit, it smolders over a particular meridian to unlock the grief that has settled there, or it readies the point to respond when the needle enters. On occasion she partly fills my navel with salt to protect its tiny pockets, and tops it up by adding moxa and lighting a match. I call out *Now* when a prickle of heat tells me it is time for her to pick the burning herb from my body. The smell and sensation of burning moxa lull me into a world away from cancer.

Always I feel comforted by her respectful and unimposing gestures. Always I look forward to my visits, to hearing her point of view and seeing the abundant and naturally tri-colored hair that frames her familiar face. There is no trendiness or judgment in her questions. She is a woman defined by her ability to listen with objective sensitivity. Wanting to share her razor perceptions and easy smile, patients return for the healing gifts that Elena offers. She is a therapist who coaxes patients to draw their own conclusion, to create their own statistic. She takes a patient's neediness and shifts it into self-sufficiency. Elena believes in the individual; everyone must look for answers within their own soul. After releasing in her company sorrows I have harbored over the years, I catch myself singing or allowing long-restrained tears to flow. I have learned to believe with Elena that freedom from fear and denial regenerates the immune system.

In the spring of 1995, the cancer clinic in Ottawa sent out a letter that noted the growing support of medical science for the use of vitamins. At my lowest ebb, during radiation and chemotherapy, and on the advice of Dr. Abram Hoffer, the psychiatrist-turned-vitamin-expert, I took sixteen grams of Vitamin C a day (far less than Linus Pauling took during his ninety-three years), lessening this dosage to five grams as the healing process took effect. In his busy office, this doctor advises cancer patients on the appropriate vitamins and dosages. He warned me against becoming tired. Habits are hard to change, and for those of us who have lived in a whirlwind, slowing down takes constant discipline. Rest, of course, allows the body time to heal itself. Most important, chemotherapy and radiation treatments put stress on the liver, kidneys, skin, and bones. A personal regime of vitamin and mineral therapies offers the immune system a velvet hand of support.

Through the clinic, I was introduced to a counselor who does therapeutic touch. I resisted the idea of counseling, having been inundated with psychological jargon during my second divorce. I went to her office reluctantly, at the suggestion of my chemotherapist. Catherine, the counselor-healer who deals with lung patients, looks younger than her years. I rolled my eyes at the friend who accompanied me. After Catherine and I had spoken briefly and I had realized the power of her intelligence, I sank back into a recliner for what I assumed would be a failed attempt to convince me of the benefits of therapeutic touch.

Catherine suggested that I shut my eyes and relax while she balanced my energy flow. I kept my eyes slightly open and watched her concentrate while she stroked the air close to my skin. Her hands moved with the grace of a butterfly, beginning at my head and moving down to my toes. As she passed over my stomach, I felt an intense warmth rise toward her hands. It was as though she had turned up my inner heater by remote control. Astonished, I looked to see if my friend's face registered the momentous event. She was studying the art on the wall. Healing without physical contact lay outside my belief; I felt respect and fear. Before I spoke, Catherine said I might feel some heat rise from my body where my energies were tangled in the ambivalence of my emotions. I kept my secret and went home stunned.

Reading up on therapeutic touch, I learned that it has gathered respect from scientists and alternative therapists for its ability to calm patients, lower their blood pressure, raise metabolism, and hasten healing. Essentially, the healer transfers *with intent* her energy to someone in need. I discovered that Catherine worked outside the clinic in a fitness center where she had a massage studio for both hands-on and therapeutic massage. I booked into her busy schedule to have both types of massage – one for aching muscles, the other for skewered emotions.

Catherine's hands know their way around the body. Often she massages a point that seems far from the pain and yet relieves it. Through hands-on massage, she enabled me to reclaim the part of myself that I never touched – my scar. When she first put a hand on my sternum, I froze. Over time, her persuasive fingers rehabilitated the untrusting sense I had of my scar tissue, making it part of the whole that is me now.

Euphoric after this in-depth massage, I fully appreciate Catherine's closing ritual – her therapeutic touch. Her hands pass so close to my body that I can feel wings of movement as she smoothes the electromagnetic field surrounding me. Her motions cool and disperse excessive energies that disrupt my equilibrium. The balance I feel afterward releases the anxiety I take to her massage table and puts in its stead a sense that all is well in my personal universe. She explained that massage and therapeutic touch are intended as preventative as well as curative: take care beforehand, and afterward takes care of itself.

This preventative approach is a major difference between traditional and complementary philosophies. Whereas traditional medicine focuses on symptom and cause after the fact of illness, complementary medicine concentrates on the interactions among spirit, mind, and body that can prevent ill health. If this interaction is not in balance, the laying on of hands smooths the bumpy road to connectedness. This balance can be scientifically calculated through physiological changes in the blood, blood pressure, and the rate of wound recovery. The extent of comfort from these therapies cannot be measured any more than a mother's love can, or a rival's jealousy. It simply and significantly changes the patient's coping powers.

To accommodate Catherine's limited availability as she moves from the clinic to her studio, I sometimes visit another masseuse. I did this reluctantly at first. Catherine had been asked to participate in restructuring the province's other cancer clinics, a feather in the cap of alternative therapies as they move into the mainstream. She would be in Vancouver for several weeks. Eventually, however, I realized that my new therapist, Jan, had her own gifts. Unlike Catherine, who stimulates me intellectually as we share our latest information on various therapies and changes at the clinic, Jan leaves me feeling I have just entered a sun-filled spa where I fall asleep to her music, my breathing synchronized to hers as it whispers into the harmony of my semi-consciousness. With dark and heavy curls flowing down her back, she brings an aura of country comfort with her presence.

On a recent visit, Jan asked if there was a particular area I would like her to work on. *Something for my nerves*, I teased her. She took me seriously. Once I was on the table, she stroked me like a cat, seeming to lengthen my arms, legs, and back without pressure. I lost track of time and place. After forty-five minutes I wobbled to my feet. *All right for driving?* she asked. *Amazing!* was all I could say. *It's called neurological stroking*, she told me as I struggled to put my foot in my shoe. At home, tucked behind the glass of a framed picture of the Greek isle of Kos, is a tiny stem of purple flowers that I picked from Hippocrates' healing garden. Inexplicably, the afterglow of massage connects me to these precious petals, and together they form a lasting metaphor for the ancient powers of healing.

Recently the Chinese martial art of Qi Gong has been introduced to North America. It motivates participants to realize the difference between the calm the body absorbs from perfecting ancient movements and the frenzy and competitiveness of modern society. Students require extensive discipline to learn its exacting demands. The process involves meditation, visualization, postures, healing sounds, and breathing patterns. Noel came with me to these four-hour classes on Saturday afternoons. We always resented giving up part of our weekend. Once there, however, we were able to discard the chaos of the week and enjoy a kind of rebirth. We returned home eager to learn the positions and to discipline ourselves to meditate for the required forty minutes a day.

For the novice, meditation takes considerable will power. Unless Noel and I did it together, we would find excuses to skip this essential part of Qi Gong. The middle-aged Chinese leader of the workshop, Hing Cheung, has the body of a youth and the enthusiasm of a child. He assures us that for every minute we meditate we add half an hour to our powers of concentration. A class member equated keeping the mind still during meditation to walking with a new puppy – one has to rein in the thoughts that bounce this way and that. Another classmate suggested we look objectively at ourselves when our minds turn to some unchangeable annoyance, to adopt a third-party viewpoint and allow the emotions to dissolve, the issue to find remedy. The instructor suggested we concentrate on our breathing and in placing the air just beneath the navel, counting breaths to keep from counting past frustrations or future deadlines.

Hing also teaches the detailed movements and healing sounds of Qi Gong. Participants station their bodies with an exact placement of hands and feet, and move their limbs either in meditative silence or with expressive sounds, focusing on the sea of life (the space below the navel), concentrating on the chi meridians (the pathways of energy), and patterning the breath to still the mind (an integral component of meditation). Each act is a move toward the perfection no one reaches. In the hours after leaving the class, students experience life as a continuing work of art.

Recent literature suggests that Qi Gong has the remarkable power to restore the seriously ill cancer patient. Knowing this, Hing gently counters the North American bias in favor of invasive treatments. He holds classes in the park in summer to lessen costs and encourage cancer patients to practice daily. Monitored studies have shown successes in both cures and lengthy remissions, for reasons that cannot be measured by traditional tools. Scientists can, however, look on the mystery of Qi Gong's achievements and be humbled.

In conversation one morning with a writer friend, I was surprised at her insistence that I visit a naturopathic physician who lives near Victoria. She was insistent that I see this physician, warning me that I should act quickly and not depend solely on conventional medicines for survival. I discovered that this naturopath, Bruce Ihara, was well-known. Getting his phone number was easy; getting an appointment meant a four-month wait. When I mentioned to his receptionist that I was being treated for lung cancer, she said she would give me the first cancellation. When she called back, I had been booked into the office in seven weeks' time.

A naturopathic physician creates and distributes homeopathic remedies. These function over time like a vaccination, a controversial form of medicine that has gained respect from people discouraged by harsh drugs, difficult surgeries, and approaches that pay little attention to diet and environmental pollutants. Naturopaths treat a patient by confronting her immune system with highly diluted natural substances that arouse a mild version of symptoms similar to those created by the disease itself. In this gentle confrontation, the immune system activates itself in the very area needed to assault a disease.

Bruce's home is an hour's drive into the countryside. His driveway winds into privacy through woods near a lake where people picnic and swim in summer. On my first appointment, he asked me to detail my medical history and eating and exercise habits. During my second visit, he tested me for allergies and other weaknesses in my body's immune-regulatory patterns. Placing a voltage meter in my right hand, a metal strip on my forehead, and my left hand in his, he took my pulses. I lay on a table as he measured my reactions, connecting me to a series of small vials and recording my pulse responses.

This bioenergetic technique is called vega testing. It works like a polygraph, monitoring skin changes as the extracts in the vials interact with electrical responses on the skin. Each extract relates to a particular organ and allows Bruce to evaluate its vitality. If an organ is found wanting, Bruce sends the patient home with remedies that encourage the organ to heal itself before the problem becomes acute, thus avoiding crisis, surgery, and expensive medicines. With each visit, at three-month intervals, Bruce reiterated that he did not believe in mega-dosing the body with any medicines, including his own, and that my health appeared to be on a slow climb to recovery, one that required vigilance without extremes.

Bruce sat on a chair behind my head while I lay facing a window with my knees raised by a bolster and my body covered with a blanket. I looked out the window on an enormous and colorful umbrella that covered women and children who danced in slow motion under its shade. The dancers moved through shafts of sunlight that stole in around the edges of the umbrella until I turned to see an elegant woman enter the office and, without speaking, place a cup of tea near Bruce. No sooner had she gone than an acupuncturist, not Elena, knelt down beside the bed table and began sharing stories full of parable and humor. I awoke when Bruce told me he had finished his examination and that I could relax while he made up my prescriptions. The dream stays with me as a message of the serenity that waits to be plumbed within the healing imagination. I had replaced the terror of morphine-stimulated images of rats and escape with subconscious blessings of communal grace.

After a year, my cancer appeared to be in remission. My chemotherapist, Heidi, shared the most recent x-rays with me, and even to my untrained eye they were noticeably clear compared to the previous ones – no tumor, no fluid, no adhesion. In her subdued way, she said the tumor was so flattened out that it was invisible. My voice faltered when I asked if this could mean the tumor was gone. She assured me this was possible and cautioned me to remain alert to changes and to return for biannual checkups. A year later, in January 1997, she suggested that I could extend my absence from six months to a year.

I have recently added Hatha yoga to my journey of recovery. I began classes in this study of *prana,* or life force, to achieve stillness of mind and balance of body. At the heart of yoga is the student's release from the outer world and increased connection to her inner one. The word *yoga* implies a union between the participant and her higher self. It concentrates on breath, our link between the inner and outer worlds. The participants in our group are people in various stages of health who eat well, exercise often, and speak softly. The instructor, Marie, small and delicate, has the flexibility of a rubber hose and the grace of a ballet dancer. She is full of surprises. Little by little I have grown to know that she is an artist who paints in summer, and a ski patrol volunteeer who maneuvers the wounded down the treacherous slopes of Mount Washington in winter. I imagined her sipping herbal tea in her garden during her spare time; instead, I have discovered that she has five children between the ages of seven and twenty. Although none of us can hope to match her youthful body or balanced postures, watching her is inspirational. We all hope that practicing yoga will inch us in the direction of the tranquillity she exudes.

Always I am rushed and distracted when I arrive because the class begins at dinner hour. With her French-Canadian accent and easy smile, Marie reads to us about the history and philosophy of yoga before we begin. We start with a sun sign, a series of postures that limber the body and that she asks us to repeat daily. The postures to follow are intended to release tensions that have built up during the week and to make us aware of our bodies and of the particular moment in time. At the end of the class, we tuck ourselves under warm blankets and follow, like dream-walkers, Marie's instructions to relax our bodies, each part in its turn, with full concentration. She wakes us with a soft, haunting chant that gradually increases our awareness. I am always grounded and energized by the time I reach home for a late dinner.

Looking back, I realize that I cannot give all the credit for my remission to either medical science or alternative therapies. I owe my being alive, cured or palliative, to the doctors and technicians who administered conventional treatments at the cancer clinic. But I owe my serenity to the alternative therapists, to their ability to engender a sense of well-being that enables me to sleep as in childhood, to awaken without incapacitating fear, to contribute to my immune response, and to be active again in my career.

As more traditional medical specialists and alternative healers join hands, more cancer patients will share in multidimensional healing. Access comes through small but growing cracks in the status quo. Complementary therapists shed light on the patient's need for the spiritual and emotional comfort that oncologists have little time to provide. In growing numbers, patients are requesting access to and funding for non-traditional treatments; slowly, the separate philosophies and practices are coming together, forced into union by genuine need.

The possibility of profound change is apparent in my acupuncturist's gentle urgings that I begin chemotherapy, my respirologist's support of an active life, my chemotherapist's belief in the power of attitude, my cancer clinic counselor's expertise in therapeutic touch, my radiation oncologist's knowledge of acupuncture, and my general practitioner's expansive awareness of complementary processes. For me, healing has come to mean a connection of flesh and feeling, science and spirit.

The daunting lung cancer statistics suggest I face a considerable challenge. And challenged patients everywhere yearn, as I did, for the magic potion that will return them to their pre-cancerous lives. But, like me, a growing number use their time and budget to seek out individualized programs of healing, common to many Europeans and Asians but still in the fledgling stage of acceptance in North America.

Just as cancer visits rich and poor alike, the disciplined and the debauched, the intelligent and the feeble-minded, so too the lottery of long-term survival falls to a mosaic of former victims. Will I be one of the blessed? I ask myself, why not? In the meantime, the Earth turns, friendships remain steady, and love carries me forward. I have become a student in the art of perfecting hope.

6

Carpe Diem

On my desk I have a small vase, so small it holds only a few blossoms. In early spring it props up a daffodil and shortly afterward a red tulip. Toward summer, I break off a sprig of lilac blossom. Mid-summer, I pluck two pansies from the shade of the cedar fence or three marigolds from the sunny deck. And when summer passes into autumn, I snip a rose from the garden. Before winter the vase carries a spray of blue florets from the puffy hydrangeas that grow near our front door. Still my favorite is the snowdrop that reminds me of winter's end, just before the purple and yellow crocuses hint of spring. Hand-painted flowers sweep around the plump center of the vase. Their blues and purples have been brushed onto a white porcelain background that rises up a slender neck and curls into a blue rim. At a glance, the vase suggests its original home in Greece and reminds me of the friend who gave it to me. *Fragile and delicate,* Skip told me. *Just like you.*

I am not as delicate as Skip made me feel, standing next to her tall body with its curvaceous hips and voluptuous breasts. Her broad shoulders could have comforted many had the need arisen. The effect of her stature was that she elicited dependence from people the way I elicit nurturing. I recall standing with her in a circle of six at a party. The three husbands were well over six feet, and the two other wives skimmed just under their size; I stood seven inches shorter than the next in line. *Damn!* I exclaimed, looking up. *I've grown so short!* Skip said, *A woman can never be too small. It's all how you call it.* She pondered a moment before she elaborated: *Fragile and delicate, that's you.* The comment was forgotten until a year later when she returned from Greece with the vase.

Skip had a largess that went beyond height. People relaxed with her because of her interest in their lives. I first met her over my second husband's and my imminent trip to Thailand. Skip invited us to see slides from her family's travels through that part of Asia. She came to the door that first night wearing an ivory sweater and red pants, her eager stride dispelling in an instant my awkwardness at entering the home of strangers. As we sipped wine and talked, I came to know her as a woman with an unwavering exuberance for sharing. Her geography lesson was the beginning of my indebtedness. To her we owed the discovery of Koh Samui with its bamboo huts and spectacular beaches, where swimming and snorkeling are as easy as waking up. She was a woman who knew how to make and take pleasure.

If I could have taken only one female friend to the proverbial desert island in the mid-1980s, I would have taken Skip. For me, she combined the stimulating joy and simultaneous relaxation of a good book. The problem was that she would have refused to come with me. She never traveled far without the man she had watched over for a quarter century. I was on the cusp of divorce when I met her, so my need for female friendship was at its pinnacle, whereas hers, in spite of her support and loyal intelligence, was nevertheless peripheral to her marriage.

At work she went by Carolyn. Big mama, big sister, big presence, she was all these in one. Although she took on the role of big sister for me, she was less than a month my elder. Yet we differed as much in the way we presented ourselves as we did in our stature. She was not a woman I would have chosen as a friend if I had let my ideals about womanhood get in the way. She bleached her hair blond, wore blue eye shadow, and painted her nails in dazzling reds and pinks, perhaps because her husband gravitated toward the gypsy in her.

I teased her about the energies she put into maintaining a look she had begun three decades before. We talked about hair dyes and make-up. My opposition probably had to do with the fact that I had tried during my marital hassles to color my hair and had created a stranger in the looking glass whose reflection made me uncomfortable. While returning to my natural silvering brunette, I simply avoided the mirror. Skip never said a word. She was not a blond who deluded herself that no one guessed, nor was she a middle-aged woman who tried to pass herself off as younger. She simply kept herself consistent with the image her husband had fallen in love with when he was nineteen. I harbored the notion that I was teaching her something about the modern woman, but I realize now that she taught me instead about the courage to be oneself. She embodied the universal and ageless nature of a woman in love with her man.

As Skip tossed a salad one evening, not long after she had been diagnosed with a melanoma and begun chemotherapy, she said, *I guess I'm going to have to stop dying my hair.* She gave me a look – *Oh well* – and began to put cutlery beside our plates. *What color will your hair be?* I asked. *I don't know,* she said. *I haven't seen my natural color for years.* For the first time in our friendship, a heavy silence filled the kitchen. *How many years?* I prodded. She thought a moment and laughed, *Since I was eighteen.* We were both within months of fifty-first birthdays, and her answer reverberated with our different pasts. She refused to be the victim of her cancer, to cry self-pitying tears or to rage against the injustice of her threatened life. Rather than denying her illness, she talked about it without losing her determination to live as long and as well as possible. She demanded that others treat her as a candidate for hope. And when this hope ran out, she continued to celebrate her life in whatever modest way she could.

The fragility of Skip's future clarified our easy connection. I knew she would leave behind a space as big as her stature. I would miss the way she looked unflinchingly at other people and interpreted their responses with originality and depth. I would miss her nonjudgmental nature, her ability to plunge with passion into every social occasion, and her generous praise of absent friends.

It seems she was better at shouldering the fears of others than in allowing others to share her own. Her home became a place where visitors could sink into the couch with a magazine, put their stockinged feet on the coffee table, and listen to the music coming from her husband's elaborate speakers, or move to the kitchen where the table overflowed with food as abundant as her appetite for life. She was always *there,* listening intently and speaking without pretense or the expectation that others would agree with her. Within her home a community of family and friends pivoted on her energies.

During the first year of my divorce, I took advantage of the pleasures that came with Skip's invitations and her *Come on in,* the phrase becoming one word when I rang her doorbell. Now that my divorce is a memory, I realize that she sustained not only her own hope but mine too when I had begun to lose faith in my ability to overcome disillusionment with men of calculating charm.

She saved her antagonism for those who hinted that her husband was not as perfect as she perceived him to be. But on two occasions when he was out of town, we changed roles and she came to my house with quivering hands and a nervous mouth. In spite of her need for comfort, she kept the sanctuary of her marriage unscathed, not disclosing the cause of her anxiety. She framed the evening with stories of their past triumphs to tide herself over the rough patches. She kept their differences sacrosanct, airing them only in his presence, never behind his back. In quarrel and adventure, he played reticent to her eagerness.

Even before my divorce I noticed how keenly she listened to my second husband as he told his fascinating stories about his theater work and our travels, and I delighted in her razor-sharp perceptions. When I went through the transition from being married to managing my social life as a single woman, Skip never excluded me. She invited me for weekend parties without trying to match me up to create an even number at the table. And during the first summer I was on my own, she asked me to drive up to their one-room cottage on Denman Island, north of Victoria.

She had rented the place for a month of summer, and I expect she knew that the drive up the Island Highway, with its glimpses of ocean between tall evergreens and outcroppings of rock, would help me to heal. With Chance in the back seat, a sleeping bag in the trunk, Keith Jarrett in the tape deck, and Skip waiting to greet me, I began to relax into my new life. When I arrived, we sat on a deck with her husband overlooking the water. The next day we walked along the deserted beach and then sought out the island's art shops. I am reminded of that summer day whenever I drink from my favorite cup, marked by a Denman Island potter with dried leaves that left a pattern of veins in the white glaze.

Skip was by nature a person who knew how to make others festive. Bit by bit, she eased me away from past wounds and into the freedom of the water's edge; I acquired new ways of seeing as we splashed in the ocean and shivered dry in the sun. She never expected me to mimic her life, simply encouraged me to trust that I would eventually find my own. I knew all the while that she would no sooner betray my secrets than she would her husband's. *Less would never be more to him*, I complained about my ex-husband's lack of appreciation for restraint. *More wasn't enough*, Skip laughed. Always her conversations circled back to me as the person responsible for my own future. I would come into her presence feeling hollow with disappointment, and leave hours later filled with an awareness of possibilities. Skip was always the first to dive into the ocean and the last to bed, and she would be there to wave me into the road as I drove into the night, alone, on my way home. I wish I could say that I wept on her shoulder, but I was not that open. In truth, I simply grumbled over her kitchen counter as she created munchies and a way for me to look at my life that differed from the one I had brought through the door. Skip became my talisman.

The mast that held up the sails of our friendship was our unwavering pleasure in each other's company, a pleasure that denied the need to compete, even when we disagreed. She was a woman who had a genuine liking for women, as she did for men, and she could talk with either sex without being defensive or flirtatious. She and I simply sailed through our experiences with the same interest in what had happened to the other as in what had happened to ourselves. None of my travels into foreign countries, movies, books, concerts, and friendships was complete until I had described the details to her and absorbed her responses. We had learned to disagree without stalling the flow of ideas or building resentments, affirming with each visit that two wrongs could make a laugh or that two rights could make a stronger argument for tomorrow.

In platonic relationships, as in love, opposites can attract. Skip and I allowed each other to grow, riding off the other's point of view. Perhaps deep friendship *is* a form of love, one that elicits the highest possibilities from the other without the jealousies of sexual connection or competition. "Each friend represents a world in us," Anaïs Nin wrote, "a world possibly not known until they arrive, and it is only by this meeting that a new world is born." The dream that Skip introduced to me brought enchantment into the frightening beauty of freedom.

When eventually I became part of a couple again, Skip's husband warned me, *Take your time, don't rush into anything.* Skip surprised me by interrupting: *You just needed someone to love you.* If anyone else had expressed this sentiment, I would have denied it after priding myself on learning to be mistress of my independence. When I introduced Skip and her husband to Noel, the first man I had taken seriously since my separation over two years before, they took to him immediately. And because he and I had a commuting relationship – alternate weekends in Vancouver and Victoria – I had lots of time in between to discuss with Skip the merits and pitfalls of allowing a man into my life again.

Against my fragile will, I listened to Skip talk about the sincerity she heard in Noel's words and saw in his blue eyes: *He hears people,* she said. *Have you noticed how he looks right at you when you're speaking with him? He's just what you need – a man without a veneer.* But I wavered: *He may just be a better actor than most.* She arched her eyebrows: *That's one way of looking at things,* she said. *At least he isn't on a mad search for a wife,* I told her. *You could probably change his mind about that,* Skip said with a grin. *Not on your life!* I said, shocked that she would expect me to consider another wedding after the sorrow of my first marriage and the fiasco of my second one, or that I would risk dreaming this man would change his perception of marriage having reached his forty-fifth birthday without having been persuaded. And so for a brief and lovely moment, I shared with old friends and a new lover the pleasures of the senses and the stories of our lives, those that had passed and those we longed to know. I suspect all of us would have said those days were happy ones.

Skip's illness had begun innocently enough, as cancer often does. Noiseless and painless, it infiltrated her life until, too late to be arrested, it had become entrenched. The word *cancer* comes from the Latin for *crab* – scuttling this way and that for survival, often hidden beneath the depths. Skip's life had begun to change when she noticed a mole on her fair-skinned torso. It matched the description of a melanoma she had read about. Her doctor told her that it was no cause for worry. But its color, size, and shape bothered her, and she returned to ask that it be removed and tested. The mole proved to be a deadly melanoma, a cancer whose cure depends on early detection; Skip's disease had already penetrated the layers of tissue to her blood stream. A specialist confirmed the diagnosis.

Too late to argue, too late to expect more than palliative treatment, Skip kept her spirits up, hoping for a miracle or determined to keep company with grace or perhaps wavering between the two. Ironically, she had trained as a nurse and was the wife of a psychologist who worked in the provincial department of health. Their knowledge of health, together with Skip's physical prowess, caused us disbelief until a cancerous tumor popped up on her breast. In a further irony, the news coincided with a similar tumor being found in her mother-in-law's breast. Each woman had the lump removed rather than the entire breast. The mother-in-law's tumor was the primary site and she went on to recover. Skip's was a metastasis, and she developed further tumors. *I'll have to buy scarves to cover my surgery at bedtime*, she told me. She said that her fair skin looked like a war zone.

Three years later, I remembered this comment when Noel convinced me that I should look at my own scar with pride. *It's a sign that you fought for your life, and I like it*, he said. *It makes you interesting.* Relieved, I soaked up his comfort, half believing him, loving him for his intent. *You're ridiculous*, I told him. *You're still here, aren't you?* he countered. How could I argue? In a misbegotten attempt to be friendly with Skip's successor, the new wife, I later revealed my scar, showing off how well it had healed and repeating the praise of my doctors and therapists for the fine clarity of the knife line. *I couldn't handle having a scar like that!* she exclaimed. I suspect she was right, and it occurred to me how well matched the new couple were. Perhaps a fear of scarring had something to do with Skip's refusing to allow the doctors to remove the lymph nodes surrounding her magnificent breasts. *There, I can relax now*, she told me in a feisty voice. *I feel as though I have some control over all the cutting that's going on.*

Skip had begun her journey by demurring in the face of everyone's sorrow when her terminal diagnosis became known. *What's all this emotion about?* she asked. *It's about affection*, I suggested. *Well, it's a bit much,* she complained, perhaps feeling as though the house were falling down around her since cancer had interfered with her capacity to do routine chores. Mistress of every nook and cranny of their home, she found herself relegated to giving orders to her husband and her twenty-five-year-old son, and watching them ignore or grapple with the housekeeping details she had established over the years.

The stress of cancer seemed to further the infrequent but regular migraines she had suffered for longer than I had known her. Migraines were another thing we had shared, and our separate medications yet another thing we discussed. Before I knew Skip, she had twice blacked out entirely, her body calling for help even then. Shortly before discovering her melanoma, she had undergone surgery for a jelly-like growth that rose up from her groin toward her waist. The doctors could not identify the substance, except to say that it was the same one that had grown back from two smaller surgeries years before. When Noel and I left to spend a month in Turkey, we convinced ourselves that Skip's headaches were normal in a patient who had undergone so many changes and such stress. But when we returned to Victoria, Skip confessed that these headaches were quite different from her migraines – constant and less intense.

We were not so much surprised as pit-of-the-stomach sad to learn that doctors had found a metastasis in Skip's brain. Her frontal lobe, the source of her personality, the essence of her self, was where a new growth had taken hold. *I'm not having it out,* she told us. *I've seen too many patients after surgery on that lobe. They sit drooling in hospital corridors, staring into space, faces blank as coconuts.* She paused to let us absorb the image and the fact that there was to be no discussion. *The doctor said I would never be the same Mrs. Morrison after the operation.* What was there to say?

Why does news of a brain tumor arouse goose bumps and shudders? Perhaps because we realize that the victim's awareness dies before her body. Although this sequence occasions more pain for the beholder than the patient, it seems like the ultimate loss of dignity. Ignorance appears blissful when others are ignorant as well. With brain cancer, the simple control we take for granted absents itself before flesh and bones cease their daily patter. The home of personhood disappears before the house that carries it, empty yet daunting.

I later learned that neither of us slept that night. She had created a more productive insomnia than I, however. She had tucked herself into her sleeping bag on the deck overlooking Finlayson Bay. All night she looked over the water and into the sky. *I've always wanted to watch the night pass into dawn and I just never took the time before,* she told me. *It was wonderful having a cold nose and warm feet.*

One evening Skip and her husband asked me to join them at a movie called *Glengarry Glen Ross,* starring Jack Lemon as a realtor who fixes the company's books to finance the medications of his seriously ill wife. The story examines the helplessness people feel in the face of private despair, the weaknesses of a man cornered by a sick wife. We stared for two hours at the dark and pathetic corners of the human soul. Skip turned to me at the end of the movie. *What did you think?* she asked. *Pretty depressing,* I said, rolling my eyes. She nodded. *I can see why people are talking about it.* Then, as we stood and began to squeeze our way toward the aisle, she collapsed in a heap. The steroids that had lessened her head pain and puffed out her upper body had weakened her legs. Her limbs had become almost ineffectual in the brief time since we had sat down. She clutched the seat in front of her, and between them, she and her husband managed to get her upright. Once standing, she was able to walk to the car. When she and I next spoke, it was on the phone. *Sometimes I wonder if I'll ever jog again,* she said in a wistful tone. *You never know*, I encouraged cautiously. She never walked unaided again in my presence.

Now, of course, I wish I had thought to tell her that memory soon diminishes the chaos of a loved one's dying. We remember, instead, when the vanished life was in full swing. I had come to realize this with my mother. Images of her as a terminal patient seldom came to mind. After a year of grieving, I thought of her as I had when my parents were centered in the heat of their lives together. But to say this to Skip, I would have had to speak of death, and we seemed to have tacitly agreed that we would talk of life instead. This included moments of anger: *They can't even bring up the laundry or buy decent bread,* she complained of her husband and son, forgetting that she had spoiled them both. *Why don't you get angry at them?* I asked. *I need them now*, she said. It occurred to me that they must have felt some anger toward her, too, as they realized how much they would have to learn to survive her absence.

In a matter of months, Skip deteriorated from the woman who complained *Don't take my role away* when I tried to help her in the kitchen, to the invalid learning to use a walker she called *that thing*, to the patient confined to a rented, adjustable bed that prevented her from sleeping with her husband. But on her final New Year's Eve, she could still use her walker to get to the couch. Noel and I surprised her and her husband with prawns, pasta, and salad while she held court from the sofa. Although her brain was cramped by the tumor, her awareness seemed sharpened rather than diminished. Her husband lit an enormous fire, and we sat around talking and munching food, forgetting for a glorious while what waited in the shadows. Skip told us that the tumor caused her to see things in repetition, like an elaborate *déjà vu*. I had been nagging Noel to sleep out on our deck since Skip had slept on hers, and now, after a glass of wine, I contemplated the joy of being able to take two runs at every event – a *déjà vu* a day.

Before Skip died, I cropped off my long hair for the first time in a decade. *Why did you do it?* she asked. *I wanted to see what I would look like,* I told her. *Come here,* she beckoned. *I can only see you with my hands now.* She capped her hands onto my head and stroked the sides of my face. *You're blind!* I whispered, as though she didn't know. Somehow she had kept it to herself, an easy secret for one as courageous as she was, made easier because she was no longer ambulatory and because we now talked more often by phone than in person. She attempted to dispel my shock: *I have always wanted to listen to the CBC and now I can do it with no interruptions.* Her tone suggested that I had no idea how to enjoy myself. When James Oppenheim said that *the foolish seek happiness in the distance; the wise grow it underfoot,* he must have been thinking of Skip. She found lilies growing in the swamp of her cancer, ones that gave off a faint perfume of hope.

CBC radio kept Skip entertained until she went deaf. Once she had lost her hearing, I felt irretrievably separated from her. The *word* coupled with the *tone* had created our friendship. She had spoken with an almost imperceptible lisp that gave femininity to her expression, a small and endearing vulnerability. Soon after her deafness set in, her husband said that the only sound she made was a deep snoring. *When it stops,* he said, *I wonder if this is it.* I could hear behind his words the longing and fear we all felt – longing for her trial to be over, fear of losing her. In little more than a year and a half, Skip had gone from an exuberant wife who had looked after her husband's every whim to a woman who could no longer sustain her own wakefulness.

Skip and I had long ago shared a book that seemed ironic

once she became ill. The title, *Hot Flashes,* is a play on the flashes women have in menopause, a passage we were both moving toward with trepidation, as women do in their mid-forties, and also a reference to the flash of recognition that accompanies new knowledge. The novel, published in 1987, a time when our friendship was solidly established and we were forty-six years old, follows a group of female friends who are forced to deal with one friend's terminal breast cancer. It ends with the fictional friends serving as pallbearers, a privilege that had previously been given to men as the stronger sex.

Back then, neither Skip nor I expected to be defeated by anything less than an earthquake or an invasion from Mars. After I had finished reading *Hot Flashes,* I sat on a stool opening a bottle of wine and arranging the hors d'oeuvre while she moved food from the fridge to the stove. *I had to bite back tears when the women were trying to keep it together,* I said. *You know, the part where their friend's body was slipping and sliding inside that damn coffin.* Skip laughed: *Did you really think they'd drop her?* A smile spread across her face. *I knew you'd like that part!* She reminded me of a sunflower – big and cheeky, its face simmering joy. Her exquisitely long fingers talked along with her words. *I didn't say I liked it exactly,* I said, and we were off again, trying to figure out what makes people notice what they do.

The fictional women made a triumphant effort to grapple with the weight of their dead friend, and the reader came to realize that the deceased had become substantial not simply in the coffin but in their spiritual lives as well. Life mimics fiction and fiction mimics life. Five years after our chatter about the book, I was at Skip's memorial service, holding up my corner of her metaphorical coffin by giving her eulogy, as family and friends held up theirs in their own ways. Skip too had become a spiritual heavyweight.

There was neither a coffin nor a body for us to carry, but we all carried her home that day.

❧

At daybreak on July 6, 1993, Skip's husband had phoned to tell me the news. It was two months before her fifty-second birthday. I hurried over and, in their bedroom, realized this was the first time I had seen a corpse before it had gone to the funeral home. When I kissed her forehead, as my grandmother had taught me to do, Skip's face was cold rubber, her features peaceful, her self evaporated. She had simply left the room without taking her body with her. In his relief and sorrow, her husband spoke of the beautiful hands that had brought him a quarter century of joy, scattering magic in the air.

Following the memorial service, family and friends had gathered with Skip's husband in the sunshine of their deck and celebrated yet another social happening at their address. I kept expecting her to appear from the sliding doors, carrying a tray of something delicious. I thought how soon the memories of a deceased person in the full steam of life replace those of her dying. In death, Skip reinforced my belief that the life spirit is a powerful force that does not die but simply takes up residence outside the body it once called home and that survivors call memory. I like to think that she knew of the people spilling out into the sunshine after her memorial service, and also of the many tears people shed at her husband's second marriage, so soon after Skip's death, when we were reminded by the similar face of her sister that she would be absent from this and all celebrations to come.

Skip had experienced times, toward the end, that would test the patience of a saint and the courage of a lioness. She once confessed that troubled people were suspicious of her opinions because she had led a blessed life, but in the end she proved that she could navigate the dark with grace and independence of thought. Swollen on steroids, she idled at death's door with her faithful cat beside her. After her husband remarried, he and his new wife sent this feline to kitty heaven when it sprayed the corners of the house to argue against the pedigreed cat that had come with another woman's baggage. Months later the pedigree developed its own cancer, beckoned perhaps by Skip's maligned companion.

A year after Skip died, I began a Ph.D., sitting in seminar rooms surrounded by students, some decades younger than myself. Although they were friendly, I felt for the first time like an outsider in the academic world. Having spent years in front of university and college classes, I had difficulty adjusting to the students' frustrations and the instructor's defensiveness. By that time, my hair had gone limp with my undetected cancer. Not yet blessed by my acupuncturist's knowledge, I was unaware that the texture of my hair was inextricably bound up with my lungs' health, linked by the same meridian. I blamed my age and became less proud of my silvering hair, especially as it hung limply beside the fading pallor of my face. When my pallor changed to fire from the fever of pneumonia, I fell asleep with damp hair and woke with strands stuck to my face and neck. Defeated by exhaustion, I realized that the long hair I had regrown that year had to be cut off again.

Eventually, I dyed my hair its original color. After the deed was done, I cheered myself by remembering the generous comments Skip had made about my once abundant hair, knowing I would have found the change in color more palatable after showing it to Skip. Her humor would have instantly changed the melancholy I felt. Sometimes I feel now that I left a portion of my innocence behind the day when, in Skip's kitchen, she faced the sudden reality of abandoning herself as a blond. No longer able to be *her* version of herself, she leapt into old age in the space of a sentence.

Skip taught me that not all people should die at home, although she would have argued the point with me. She told me stories of ways in which her son had been forced to help her, prompting him to acts of intimacy from which she, as a mother, would have preferred to shelter him. Friends had complained that they could not visit with ease because they feared disrupting the privacy of husband and son, although I had always been made to feel welcome. Dying, it seemed to me, would come more easily to those who do not have to worry about being an encumbrance in the house where they once played mistress to its needs. Perhaps, too, a patient should be able to grieve for her own dying without feeling responsible for the inconvenience to others. But what exhausted family can make a decision that may seem a betrayal of a loved one? And what dying person can make that decision for herself when home is the ultimate sanctuary?

According to Skip's husband, she spoke to him just once about her dying. She did not talk of herself. Instead she asked him, *What will you do if I don't make it?* He said, *I'll manage.* We soon learned that he spoke the truth. When we arrived at his house for dinner a few weeks after the wake, we were surprised to find a stranger, a woman our age, putting Skip's dishes on the table. The atmosphere grew dense with awkwardness. After a glass of wine, I demanded to see Skip's wardrobe and left the house in her enormous sunbonnet. I can hardly explain my taking it except to say that when I looked in the bedroom and saw that her clothes and medications had not yet been removed and that a stranger had slipped in among them, I felt compelled to safeguard her dignity.

Each of us simply did what we had to do as we bumbled through the process of getting on without Skip. *I think I'll arrange for someone to clean out my private stuff after I die,* I told Noel, peering out in the dark from under the floppy brim. *Don't worry your head about that,* he said. Skip's hat, a tailored bonnet with blue and pink flowers, dwarfed me, and it eventually came to remind me of that final dinner with an innocent stranger who had been made to feel unwelcome by Skip's friends. Within months, she was replaced by a less innocent woman who led Skip's widower to the altar and out of town. I last saw him sporting an earring and heading toward the Okanagan.

When Noel and I married, Skip's widower did not come to our wedding. *People change,* Noel consoled me. *You're not kidding,* I agreed. *Look at us,* he coaxed. I couldn't argue. We were gathering that settled feeling in our bones that neither of us had thought was possible again. Noel had helped me to weather Skip's death, and his nurturing would be a prelude to his imaginative care during my own confrontation with cancer. The dreams that we two couples had once shared were irretrievably changed by the lightning jolts of Skip's death and my illness.

In time, I gave the hat away. Skip had returned to her primal beginnings in the sea, and I had all I needed from her – her example of how to leave behind an undiminishing example of courage. A friend's dying is both a loss and a gift. We become wiser, more humble. Sorrow cannot be separated from beauty, from the remembrance of times that made a difference – the Christmas when I was alone and she invited me to share dinner with her family and friends, or the Friday night she went to a church concert because I was part of the choir, or the delicate brass tuning bells she ordered for my birthday so I could find my vocal note without the piano, or the many times I woke covered with a blanket after falling asleep during a video. Skip haunts me even now to remember the rewards of cherishing small and daily gifts, of making adventures of the past and energy of the future.

Women are forever being reminded to stand up for themselves in society, an ability that came naturally to Skip. Even in the extremes she would go to in her effort to please her husband, she made clear that she was doing so from desire and self-esteem, not fear or self-deprecation. Through trusting her I came to trust myself and to learn the reality in the old saying that to have love, you must offer it. Skip's intelligence had been as versatile as it was formidable, although she had never bothered to acquire academic credentials, as so many in her circle of friends had done. Hers was a knowledge that came from innate wisdom fleshed out by working as a mental health nurse. She had too much fresh air in her soul to spend years in the musty archives of university libraries, looking for truths that can be found in the eyes of living people. Spreading light wherever she moved, Skip was asked her opinion even into her dying days.

Her doctor, for example, realized her ability to see beyond textbook answers. Like all of us, he brought his stories to her for a bedside opinion because she was never self-indulgent, never one to use tears or maudlin comments to elicit sympathy, never given to blaming past cruelties. One night, the doctor talked with her about the Rollerblade gangs that were raising a storm outside his medical office. Those who leased offices in the complex had met to discuss the problem, but their resolve to stop the teen-agers from inflicting danger on the slower patients and caregivers had no effect except to frustrate those who were more mature and less agile. On the day of such a meeting, the doctor sat down on the bed next to hers and told her all the details. *Is everyone represented at the meetings?* she asked. *Most of us*, the doctor answered. *What about the kids?* Skip suggested. *The kids!* he exclaimed, as though someone had just illuminated the night.

Where is Skip's light now? I want to know whether her ashes were swept back into the sea with the rising tide to become fodder for other lives. I want her to know that she reveals herself to me in the purple and blue florets I snipped from a hydrangea blossom on a recent autumn morning. These four-petaled flowers spill over the edge of my Greek vase, speaking to me in the November moment while the earth tilts toward the darkest part of the year. *Carpe diem*, they say to me, *seize the day* – the message of the ephemeral flower.

Those who loved her remain part of the floral season that was Skip. When I see myself through her reflection, I am no longer an ordinary woman. Because of my cancer and in spite of it, I have become a woman who knows the preciousness of each passing day and that each kindness, no matter how small, lives on in the lives of others. These are the petals of a friendship lost to the earth but not to the soul.

7

Farewell Kathleen

I met Kathleen Ryan during a tennis match she organized for college faculty in the fall of 1991. Neither of us knew we had cancer, although the clinic later assured us the disease had hunkered in our lungs for at least a decade before making itself known. Otherwise, I knew Kathleen only by reputation. She was the warrior queen of the faculty association, challenging people she had decided were morally feeble and self-serving, those whose opinions she considered to be a hindrance or irrelevant, and faculty who allowed their egos to overshadow a democratic decision. Unlike Skip, Kathleen stood barely five feet tall. Yet she made grown administrators tremble when they offended her idea of justice, and others grateful when she argued passionately on their behalf.

We did not speak again until we were on the same side of the net in a match against cancer. I phoned her one year after she had been diagnosed; I had just been told I had a lung tumor and I wanted to commiserate. I wonder now if we were in any way affected by our cancers that night of tennis. My 1992 x-rays to probe the cause of severe chest pain had come back negative, but I did not know then how little even the trained eye can detect in the light and shadow of x-rays. Were Kathleen and I tired by mutant cells feeding on the abundant pulmonary blood vessels that make lung cancer so formidable? Had her left lung already begun to collapse? Cancer is sneaky. It often comes slowly and with little pain, defeating its victims as they try to accommodate what appear to be common signs of early middle age – lessened energy and aching bones. We begin to hurt, as Leonard Cohen says, in the places where we used to play.

After my diagnosis, when the doctors advised me to avoid fatigue, I promised myself and Noel I would ignore unessential pressures. But I found this simple goal as hard to attain as it is to change any lifetime habit in a world where the quest for stimulation often replaces the human need to enjoy the process. For a while I thought of *tired* as a natural state. I remind myself now to turn homeward with the goal of finishing my walk, cycle, or paddle before I deplete my energy. Inadvertently, I discovered through this change that sleep comes more easily when the immune system still percolates, when bedtime arrives before exhaustion.

Cancer, after all, speaks of a point where natural immunity has broken down, allowing cancer cells to enter a heyday of exponential multiplication. It also speaks of death unless the rapid and disorderly imbalance can be arrested. A person's immune system is her best friend, and it needs to be nurtured to remain at the ready. Perhaps rest knits up the raveled sleeve not only of care but also of cancer, and the return to balance defines remission.

I did not see Kathleen's face again until almost four years after our tennis match when she visited me after my surgery. With her she had two gifts: a container of yogurt and a community health nurse and friend, Carolyn. The nurse had brought with her a special pillow to ease the discomfort of my newly severed chest. She would subsequently rescue me from dehydration and the clogged bowels that accompany drugs for pain, and from the sunstroke that I had brought on by driving down the highway with an open sunroof. Just prior to this visit, Kathleen had introduced me by phone to the idea of visiting her acupuncturist, Elena. Of all my friends' gifts, Kathleen's sharing of Carolyn and Elena were offerings I could not have managed without during my initial struggle to regain my life.

As I came to know Kathleen, I realized how little we had in common beyond our mutual diagnosis, our ages, and the college where we taught in our separate departments. She had spent her early life struggling with clinical depression, whereas I had not known unhappiness until I confronted the disillusionment that precedes divorce. If left to acknowledge her own body clock, Kathleen woke up when I was contemplating lunch, and I went to bed just as she was becoming engrossed in her books and letter writing. During her radiation, when her concentration was hampered by distress, she found relief by watching television, whereas I felt lonely at the thought of watching daytime shows, and I spent my daylight hours walking and reading or, when I was able, writing these stories.

Kathleen once surprised me by saying she had been unable to remove the small bandage that covered her exploratory incision that revealed she was inoperable. As a member of our union executive, she could speak with articulate humor or anger to a crowd of opinionated faculty. I took a deep breath one morning after a shower and removed the bandaging that had covered my neck-to-navel surgery. Yet I had taken years to speak at small meetings, where the beating of my heart had silenced me. Kathleen, as well, confessed she felt jealous of the doctors' decision to risk surgery on me and to offer me chemotherapy in conjunction with radiation. Her jealousy quickly flew out the window, she said, when she discovered that the surgeon had sawed through my sternum before realizing I too was inoperable. Since then three other women − a friend at

Whistler, another colleague at the college, and a high-spirited woman in publishing – have each had a lung tumor successfully removed with its surrounding lobe. My reaction was unconditional joy because I felt somehow that good news is contagious and that I might possibly be on a roll with them, a roll toward survival. Perhaps mine is a self-centered interpretation of the biblical passage about casting bread upon the water and having it return tenfold.

Kathleen was able to talk and write easily about her fear of death. I leaned toward the Eastern philosophy that fear opens a door for death to enter; when I speak of it I feel as vulnerable as I do if I confront the gods by daring to consider myself cured instead of in remission. (Perhaps the word *remission* does not seem as harsh to me as it does to others since my own mother gained years through its blessings, and my former father-in-law remained in remission for nearly thirty years.) Different as we were, though, Kathleen helped me enormously by introducing me to a crucial support system and to intelligent literature on cancer. Perhaps most important in our connection was that, initially, we were the only people we knew who shared our disease and so we could understand each other's boundless interest in the topic.

After we had compared reactions to our cancer, our doctors, and our treatments, we agreed that living close to nature and in the moment are two ways for cancer patients to lessen their fears. Nature invites a spiritual comfort that brings acceptance. Being in the moment provides an opportunity to make each day a work of art. Kathleen's ocean deck offered a feast for the eyes, a parade of nature at its living best, a distraction full of meaning. It enticed her to take an all-women sailing cruise. Similarly, my home is within minutes of the Strait of Juan de Fuca, where I can look across to the Olympic Mountains on my morning walks.

For me, kayaking became an invaluable form of meditation. Knowing that water always wins, I remained alert while paddling or storing my kayak, or setting up camp above the tide line for the night. Nature's simplicity forced me to forget my fear of metastasis as I bathed in the cold water or washed my dishes at its edge. Just as nature quickened my body, it slowed my mind, sucking me into a vortex of thought untainted by loneliness, making me aware that all living things, not just the ailing, thrive temporarily. I began to realize I was both common and unique, lasting and finite.

Noel and I rented an ocean kayak and set out for five days with four other people to explore the shorelines around the Gulf Islands between Victoria and Vancouver. Negotiating tides and undercurrents, struggling against crosswinds, I was mesmerized by the dip and rhythm of my paddle. At times I simply gazed at sky, land, and water, relaxing into my small, seemingly safe place in the universe. We watched the wildlife going about its daily business of survival – an eagle perched on a rocky island, still as a pyramid, watchful and unflinching; baby seals on the rocky thrusts of land, their lactating mothers splashing about to distract us, the large males bobbing around the kayaks; and mountain goats on the rock face, their agile offspring bounding up vertical inclines. The expansive landscape allowed me to tap into a vast well of inner space, my thoughts drifting toward a need to maneuver myself from tragedy to challenge.

During one of my visits to the cancer clinic, I was surprised to see Kathleen and Carolyn leaning against a wall while the nurses sorted out a confusion in appointment times. Kathleen fretted while she waited for her x-ray results on her one-year anniversary of radiation treatments. My treatment differed considerably from hers for a variety of reasons: my lung had not collapsed; my cancer was in the right upper lobe rather than the larger left one; I had endured serious surgery; and my tumor appeared to be closer to the mediastinum than hers was. She had not been given the chemotherapy I was about to undergo in conjunction with radiation. At that moment, I wondered why she would feel so frightened of her x-rays when she seemed to be recovering. The following year I understood perfectly the terror of waiting to hear a doctor's words that would either send me home free for six months or back to the hospital a captive. I waited for Kathleen to phone with her results. When she did not, I feared the worst and phoned her. I interrupted her celebrating a healthy x-ray, and she expressed surprise and gratitude at my concern.

During my convalescence, Kathleen visited my home. We talked over spinach pie and tea about our favorite bible of cancer therapies, a book by Michael Lerner called *Choices in Healing*. Kathleen researched the literature on her cancer as one would a Ph.D. thesis topic, whereas I rested my mind in order to connect with my body. That afternoon she asked if I would go to Common Weal with her, an institution that Lerner runs in California, where people go for help in coping with a terminal diagnosis. In spite of my failed surgery, daunting statistics, and the fact that I was mid-treatment, I had not dwelled on being terminal except when I allowed myself to grow overtired. But I agreed to accompany her if she wished to go. When she did receive her final diagnosis, however, she decided to create her own *un*common weal with her partner Michael. They spent the summer counting whale sightings from the glorious deck he had built. As capable with stove and washer as he is with saw and hammer, he made Kathleen's days slip by without unnecessary strain or deprivation. She wrote in her diary, *I can always cry if Michael is there.*

When Kathleen was diagnosed with metastases, I was the last of her friends to know. Each time I called, she and Michael managed to keep their secret from me, and people at the college never mentioned that her abdominal pain and cough had been diagnosed in April, by ultrasound, as the spread of her primary cancer. On a brief trip to Massachusetts, I was suddenly struck as I wandered through an art gallery by the possibility of Kathleen's being ill. When I returned home, I confronted Michael and he told me that before I had boarded the plane, Kathleen had indeed been rushed by ambulance to the city and had almost died from an allergic reaction to chemotherapy. She had then suffered from many of the side effects I had been so fortunate to avoid. A mutual friend later confessed that Kathleen had specifically asked that I *not* be told. She did not want me to wonder if her new diagnosis would eventually be mine.

I walked around numb for two days before Kathleen and I renewed our telephone friendship. After an initial awkwardness, we chatted about many things: her chemo-related heart problems and damaged hearing, the newly published literature on cancer, the fact that her hair was growing back, and her complaints about people who came uninvited and allowed their children to make havoc of her home and peace of mind. She talked of resting late in the luxury of her upstairs bedroom and of thinking about the spirit of the ocean washing over her. She wrote lists that compared the hospital to the home as a place to die, with home the winner. There she could hear the cat snore, watch the sun from her bedroom window, and smell the wind off the water. She listed, too, the ways in which she was able to be herself in the lack of formality that home allows, to whine and grump and still be loved, to hear no questions about bowel movements or enemas, and to have a final and sacred ritual without the need to ask permission or to include an unwanted audience.

Kathleen and I had lunch near the end of her life, and the memory of that day fills me with regret. We were on the balcony of a restaurant in Sooke, an hour's drive from Victoria. Oddly enough, as we sat drinking herbal tea and eating fruit pie laden with ice cream, our talk seldom touched on death. Our more immediate problem was to avoid swallowing the wasps that threatened to enter our mouths with each forkful. As she batted at the wasps, I had to push away thoughts of George Orwell's story about a man being led to the gallows who avoids a pool of rainwater. The author marvels at the man's desire to keep his feet dry minutes from the end of his life. I resisted this thought because I had unwittingly resisted the knowledge that Kathleen's final days were approaching. I wanted her to stay alive, to buffer me from further loss.

And as we ate and shooed wasps, I would not entertain the thought that she would actually die, even though she attempted to share her vision of imminent change. If I were to explain my resistance, I would have to say that she did not smell of death or have the haunted look I have seen in the faces of others close to death. She was still mobile, opinionated, and breaking diet rules. But she sought my acknowledgment of her pending death; she wished to roll the concept over in our conversation and to study its repercussions and my reactions. She wanted me to accept her for what she was – a woman dying in early middle age. Dying is a lonely undertaking, and perhaps she simply wanted someone to recognize the immensity of her task.

I would not or could not accept her truths that day. She worried, for example, that after her death Michael would perhaps find the wrong woman to keep him company. I told her I would not want Noel to remain alone after all he had done for me. Knowing that Michael had done as much in his own way for Kathleen, I hoped my words would discourage her from causing him future guilt. On the surface my point seemed valid, but later I recognized my error. What woman who has loved a man would not feel saddened at the idea of becoming a memory, however cherished, especially if her illness had caused their connection to blossom, and more especially if they had grown to realize its preciousness through the limitation of time? Kathleen's vision had reached deeper than my own, and I later realized that I could not contemplate with equanimity the idea of any woman making Noel's face light up as I can do when we greet each other to begin a new day, or of some other woman hearing the click of the gate when he comes home.

When Kathleen had unexpectedly metastasized to her liver, kidneys, and adrenal glands, she kept diary notes on the process of dying. *So soon, so soon,* she wrote upon learning that her liver tumor was growing again and that the recent chemotherapy treatment meant to arrest the tumor had reached the end of its promised life extension. Our chemotherapist had told us both that the treatment raises a major problem when it does not kill off *all* the errant cells. Remaining cells that have proven themselves too strong to be eradicated, once restored, return with a vengeance.

Kathleen's dying caused her to question conventional choices. She was adamant, for example, about refusing a second series of chemotherapy treatments, and with it another possible extension, because of the chemicals' debilitating effects on her heart and hearing. I argued that she should extend her life at all cost, throwing in the cliché that where there is life there is hope. It did not occur to me that my belief, like her own, was predicated on an individual response to chemotherapy. Instead, I loaned her a book by Reynolds Price, who tells of the timely invention of a scalpel that allowed doctors to remove a hefty part of his formerly inoperable spinal cancer, and to save his life. When she quarreled with me over the lunch bill, I snatched it up and jauntily treated us. Later I realized that she had wanted to share, to hold her own as death withered her grasp on life, or simply to give after having received so much from attentive friends.

She wrote again in her diary, one week after our lunch when a visitor came to proselytize about his religious belief, *I feel often the visitor waits to hear something from me, some pearl of wisdom, some insight. I have none. . . . Dying is lonely, but I need time to be alone; I need time to be lonely.* I went through this section of her diary nervously, expecting to find myself criticized, and I was relieved to find that she had been more patient with me than I had been with her. I had lacked the wisdom to relieve the loneliness of her dying; I was not perceptive enough to allow her to express her own contradictions and contemplative truths.

Reading about Kathleen's rejection of frequent visitors reminded me of my own initial diagnosis. I was unable at first to relate to anyone but Noel because our grief knew no words. He rocked me gently, body against body, as our burden of shock and fear subsided, and I was gradually able to accept the disappointment and challenge, to map out with his help a new life. I remember looking forward to bedtime – sometimes simply moving from the couch to the bedroom – not because I was tired or amorous, but because I felt a childlike security in the privacy of his arms. I suspect Kathleen felt a need, as I did, to escape the faces of people struggling to make her happy and to make themselves comfortable. Few people, whether victim or observer, can avoid shock and discomfort in the presence of a terminal diagnosis. *Awesome,* with its dimensions of meaning, describes the emotion that often surrounds the word *cancer.* Both visitor and patient seem awed by the prospect of acknowledging death, the only event as common as birth.

At the end of the afternoon, when I drove Kathleen home from the restaurant, we sat in the car talking about her prognosis. I told her I had something to offer that I wanted her to take seriously. She interrupted: *You mean you know I am going to die?* I waved off her courageous overture with a smile, saying with the authority of the ignorant, *We were just stuffing ourselves with pie and wasps!* I assumed she had risked an indulgence, an adventure of sorts, because she felt sure enough of recovery to afford one. I then offered up our guest room for overnight stays if she and Michael had to come into the city. She did not meet my eyes when she said, *Oh, thanks.* She said she had been given nine weeks to live and had already used up three of them. Looking at the small face that peered out from under her white sailing hat, I said that I could not see her as a dying person. In fact I grew so enamored by my idea of her survival, so dependent on *my* need for her to survive, that I suggested we celebrate the year 2000 together.

By comparison, I realize, Noel allowed me to know without words that he would be there for me whatever the road, that I did not have to pretend I was well if I was not, that instead we had to do what was necessary to regain peace of mind and, possibly, my health. My brother-in-law, Ken, a friend of more than twenty-five years, responded to my illness simply by saying he was sorry this was happening to me. His face spoke his grief, and he did not presume to know what my future would be or to replace my thoughts with his own. My sister, Lynne, massaged me with body oils, having learned from hospice the importance of touch.

Kathleen and I did not hug good-bye in spite of having hugged hello. I suspect that I opposed anything that might imply finality. When she climbed out of my car, I longed to rush after her, but I wondered, like Prufrock, if this would be excessive, if a hug would appear to be more than the warmth of one woman to another, one cancer patient to another. Instead, I waved as I turned onto the highway and yelled out the window, *I'll call you.* She walked through her garden gate and I never saw her living face again.

I did, however, hear her voice. A week after our lunch I called to say I wanted to return her book and pick up one I had loaned her. With a softer voice than usual, she suggested that I pass it to someone else in need. As I listened to her cough, I hoped there was time enough to hear her become cheeky again, to listen to her denounce her favorite enemies at the college and praise Michael for his support.

Kathleen learned from Elena about a program called SOPHIA, the Greek word for *wisdom.* The acronym stands for the Study of the Philosophy of Healing in Action, and two lines from a classical Chinese poem by Lao Tzu-Tao Teh Ching express the promise of this program: *What is well planted cannot be uprooted. / What is well embraced cannot slip away.* After her diagnosis, Kathleen had driven down to Seattle to immerse herself in four intensive weekend workshops on how to access this healing. Its premise involves the pursuit of balance through new perceptions. The search for health begins by comparing classical Chinese thought with modern

Western ideas to enable students to gain new awarenesses of their behavior and attitudes and to acquire knowledge through contrast. Goethe suggested this method of seeing through comparison when he wrote, *To know only one language is to know no language.*

Students are asked to pattern their thoughts in accordance with the cycles of nature, to move through the circle of seasons with an awareness of change. Participants learn to translate nature's passages into personal ones and, in doing so, to acquire the self-knowledge that leads to a balance between feelings and actions. In time, they learn to respond more productively in direct proportion to their abilities to listen more keenly, to hear more than superficial words of communication, and to observe without judgment their own lives and others'. By taking time to observe the self, each student begins to move away from stress and pain, to enter into harmony and peace. SOPHIA defines life as a rice pot on simmer, a combining of elements to create sustenance. Kathleen said this was the single most important acquisition in her final year. When she described SOPHIA to me, she credited it with teaching her the hardest thing of all, to accept the truth of her own unique being.

When a mutual friend phoned to save me from hearing about Kathleen's death through our faculty voice mail, I was grateful and saddened. I was also surprised. My father had taught me that failure happens only when a person stops trying. Over the years I had translated this to mean that a person is not to be counted out until the natural processes of the body are silenced; in the meantime, I should not give up moving one foot in front of the other on behalf of others or myself. My surprise told me that I had not lost hope for Kathleen in spite of all that had gone before my phone rang.

In her passing, Kathleen left me forever changed. I had wanted to believe that death comes with ample warning. Not the medical alerts, but the intuitive ones that make the eye look inward and the body turn away. I wanted to know that I could trust my reflection in the mirror to tell me when my remission was over. I reasoned that a dying person must be visibly helpless, frail, or frightened, especially when the cause of death is cancer. Otherwise I would not have time to clean out my closets and drawers, to tell Noel what a miracle of joy and confidence he had brought into our shared days, to tell my friends how each had added to my life, to tell Lynne that after our river of difference had widened to an ocean, I did not know how to reach her any more than she knew how to reach me. The expression *untimely death* took on new meaning.

Kathleen had not waited for the disease to take away her strength before she put her emotional and intellectual house in order. In spite of her committed relationship, her home overlooking the water, and her career, she opened herself to death with a grace and stamina that allowed her, ironically, to extend her active life rather than foreshorten it. Unlike the clichés for the dying that Carol Shields mocks through her long-suffering protagonist in *The Stone Diaries*, Kathleen went into a rapid decline just twenty-three hours before her final breath. I imagined her asking the Grim Reaper to stop lurking around and to climb into her bed and share the designer sheets she had bought to soothe her way.

By example, Kathleen taught me about the dignity of knowing when the battle is over, when elegance is found in acceptance rather than struggle, when the time has come for the final voyage. Although she and I cannot be together in flesh, she speaks to me, as I read her diaries, of her longing to be understood, of her fear of the unknown, and of her growing acceptance. I am given a blessing, a second chance to acknowledge her message and to say a humble farewell. In her last days, Kathleen did not lose hope. She simply changed it to encompass a way of dying. As a couple, she and Michael taught me the difference that a responsible and devoted partner can make for a person trapped in the irrevocable stage of remission, and showed me that a cancer patient who has moved beyond the possibility of recuperation can still retain hope, not for a miraculous recovery but for a dignified and meaningful death.

A friend who came from San Francisco to help Michael organize the memorial service noticed Kathleen's father's watch on the windowsill in the bathroom. When she inherited the watch, Kathleen had replaced the wristband and begun wearing it. After her final diagnosis in early August, however, she had refused to wear any timepiece, a gesture to the importance of her own moments as opposed to linear time. The watch had been left to sit on the sill, its unseen hands offering a premonition. The hands had stopped at 9:45 P.M., the time of Kathleen's last breath on the night of September 24, 1995.

This mysterious connection between life and death, between what has been and what is, brought to mind a poem written by Gwendolyn MacEwen before her death at the age of forty-six. In *Dark Pines Under Water*, she wrote of the superficial and the subconscious, of connectedness between spirit and intellect, of Canadian nature and the explorer's astonishment, of the mysteries shrouding life, and of the writer's struggle to define them: *And you become a forest in a furtive lake; / The dark pines of your mind reach downward / ... In an elementary world; / There is something down there and you want it told.* A terminal diagnosis takes the patient into an elemental world where she must discover her own unique landscape of mortality.

True to herself to the end, Kathleen had demanded to be allowed a funeral where people could gather in a small chapel by the sea at the edge of her village. The bishop overrode the village priest's objection, agreeing that all Catholics, in spite of their absence from mass, are welcome to the rituals that take place within the stucco sanctuary with its wooden steps and peaked roof. Having arranged what she could and trusting Michael with the rest, she climbed without assistance a flight of stairs to their bedroom and died. The life force of Kathleen Ryan spent itself within the walls he had built for them, and in the presence of those who loved her.

One of our colleagues, Moira Walker, wrote a poem that she dedicated to Kathleen and read at her memorial service. It's called *Coming to Life.*

It is apt that Michelangelo's creator,
    leans lovingly forward to touch
        his departing Adam
          one last time.
    (Were the painting mine, it is true,
    I'd connect the two more closely.)
What initiates life is caress-borne:
    The cow licks the calf to standing;
    Beak meets beak as adult feeds those
        too young to fly;
    Hens brood their eggs awake;
    Seeds swell as surrounding peach begins to grow.
Nothing survives that has not
        been warmed at another's side.
Why then voice surprise
    when the doctor-healed youth turns physician,
    when the gently prodded pupil becomes teacher,

when the tenderly raised child assumes the
parent's path.
No, not what twists in our genes,
but the timely thought,
the heartfelt glance,
the departing touch
determines our engagement.

We come to life through others. I suspect that if I have learned
more ways than I once knew about how to befriend a person who
faces death, these lessons took hold upon coming to know
Kathleen, and then hearing this poem.

Like Kathleen's diaries, Michael's pictures record the world
she left us to share. He showed me a photo he took shortly before
she died. Immersed in the hot tub on their deck, she is laughing
into the sun, her hat pulled down to shade her eyes. The face
Michael has caught is full of affection and mischief. Together they
have locked in place their own substantial farewell, their moment.
But the picture I love best was taken before Kathleen's diagnosis.
It is of Michael with his thumbs hooked into the suspenders that
hold up his blue jeans. His eyes, dark and bright, suggest surprise
and laughter. He wears the look of a man who has conquered his
own small corner of the universe. Kathleen stands behind him, snug
against his back, her arms around his waist. She wears the impish
grin that all who have known her remember and love. It suggests
she has caught someone worth catching.

On the day of her funeral, a breeze carried the message of
autumn. Floating leaves wandered through the afternoon sunshine,
reminding everyone of the constancy of change. Inside Saint Rose
of Lima Catholic Church, a black and white photograph of
Kathleen greeted the family, friends, and colleagues who gathered

there. In profile, she looks into the distance, a gentle smile on her lips, her gaze thoughtful.

I am left with a keen sense that she has become a part of the ocean's light now, that she continues to make us see the landscape with a deeper appreciation of its beauty. She, who never considered herself an artist, has painted the water and trees of Sooke in new shades. Since her death, my moments in nature have been enhanced by a repeated and spontaneous acknowledgment of a woman who enriched my definition of dying. I listen clearly to her now. I have learned that *farewell* does not always mean *good-bye*. There is an old Norse definition that precedes *good-bye* and translates into *travel well*. And so I find myself saying *fare well* to my comrade in cancer as she meanders through the lives of those she touched.

When Michael spoke at Kathleen's service, he said the luck of summer had brought them more whale sightings than either could remember, and a spectacular moment one dusk when they heard a sharp exhale, and saw the glisten of a dorsal fin. They had carved out time to explore the passing tales of water, to plumb the depths of friendship. He spoke, too, of how Kathleen had compared herself to a guest on a cruise liner, luxuriating from her deck chair in the simple and dependable pleasures of rising and falling waters. He left his listeners with an image of Kathleen happy and safe on the wooden deck that ends where the cliff begins its sharp descent into the sea.

8

Light It from Mine

Love is the damnedest thing. It slants into corners unexpectedly, as the sun does when it angles across the garden. Its warmth makes even the most unlikely plant burst into flower. A few years after my second divorce, that culprit, happiness, began to invade my spirit in ways I had almost forgotten. Love poems began to make sense again, I smiled at strangers, got teary-eyed in movies when the hero met the heroine, and repeatedly told Chance how much I loved her. We are supposed to reach an age when we learn the benefits of moderation in all things, but this does not seem to come easily in matters of the heart. And so just before I reached fifty, I fell in love again. And just as in a silly movie, I fell for the boy next door.

Well, he wasn't really a boy anymore, but a forty-five-year-old man. Noel wasn't even the man next door, but he had been some years before. We seemed to share the usual feelings of people alone in mid-life – a disbelief that love could come knocking hard enough to wear down the apprehension that grows with experience, and a longing to be understood and understanding with a committed friend. As well, there was the yearning to touch and be touched within the sanctuary of private affections – the powerful beast was not hobbled by age as I had assumed as an embarrassed teen-ager that it should be.

Dating, as single people over forty know, has little of youth's innocence but much of its awkwardness and boredom. Each time I went out with someone new, I swung from apprehension to apathy, thinking often about something I was reading or the comforts of my privacy. I preferred to spend my time with married couples and to avoid the discomfort of easing out of something I should not have entered in the first place. Nothing in my daily life gave me reason to hope that I would again find someone with whom I could willingly share my appetites and interests, but the heart has its own agenda. The small voice of childhood sang of my father when my guard was down. But after a year on my own, I had learned to submerge these wistful longings under a tidal wave of activities.

Before he moved to Vancouver, Noel lived next door to my second husband and me in Victoria. I knew little about him except that he owned the cooperative house where many people lived in apparent harmony that revolved around Noel's cousin, a brilliant, beautiful, handicapped woman of my age who looked after Chance while I taught. Noel always seemed to be leaving to work on his thesis or attend some political meeting whenever I visited their round oak table, a place where family and friends entertained one another from noon until midnight. Gossip had it that Noel had had his heart broken years before and that he had subsequently been with a woman noticeably younger than himself. During my conversation with this young woman, in which we confessed to our unhappinesses in our current relationships, she told me that Noel was not an easy man to pin down. I thought how wonderful that would be, as my second husband could be pinned down by just about any woman with an appealing smile.

With this scanty knowledge, I was surprised – long after my

divorce, and after his cousin's death – when Noel invited me to hear Bob Dylan at the Pacific Coliseum in Vancouver. Since the last ferry returned to Victoria at 9 P.M., I would have to stay overnight. I packed Chance's dog food with my flannelette nightie and arrived at Noel's house for a Saturday afternoon at Granville Market, a night at the concert, and a Sunday preparing for September's lectures on the ferry home. Not having mentioned that I'd been to two Dylan concerts in my younger years, and having no idea why Noel would think I liked folk music, I wondered if he might be a little presumptuous. Neither did I tell him that at the first concert my second husband and I had sat close enough to Dylan (with The Band in Seattle) to count his lip wrinkles, nor that someone in a row above me had thrown up over my long hair when he later visited Vancouver. I had relegated my infatuation with Dylan to my counter-culture days that had ended when the 1980s began. On the ferry to Vancouver I remembered that it had been a long time since I had done anything I didn't want to do in order to be with a man, especially one who made me feel like an intellectual wasteland.

I suspect that our pre-concert dinner at a small Italian restaurant near the university surprised us both. Perhaps it was the jazz pianist who charged our batteries. Perhaps this first date was the seed that flowered into a colorful autumn. *How did that compare to your other rock concerts?* Noel asked on the way home. *It was quite good,* I lied. *How about you?* He looked a little sheepish before confessing that he had never been to a rock concert before. *But you played your guitar all the time you lived next door,* I said, bewildered. *Not really,* he said, embarrassed that I remembered. *Mouth organ too. Just like Dylan,* I insisted. *Think you must have been imagining things,* he said. We walked around Point Grey where he lived outside the gates of the university. *Heavy perfume really turns me off,* he said as we admired the natural perfumes of late summer in the neighborhood gardens. *It ruins a lot of nights at the opera, trying to see the stage through watering eyes,* I agreed. *Maybe some men need kick-starting like old cars,* I added, compelled to defend foolish women. We laughed as we turned up his walk, but I refused to look at him when I went off to my separate bedroom and snuggled down, Chance on the floor beside me. The next morning, we ate breakfast to classical music in a lovely café before we enjoyed the sunshine of Stanley Park. When I left to catch the ferry home, we gave each other a shy hug. It seemed odd that I should feel energy on a man whom I had not yet kissed, yet I was unable to do anything more than look out over the water and think of clever things to say next time we met.

A few weeks later, when Noel returned from Vancouver to organize a communal garage sale, say good-bye to his tenants, and empty his house for the new owners, we spoke briefly. I asked if he would like to join me and friends for dinner, and as an aside I told him he could stay the night if he was too late to catch his ferry. *I have a tiny guest room,* I told him. *It's in the basement but it's solid cedar, like sleeping in a hope chest,* I teased. *Is it the servants' quarters?* he asked. *It could be if you want to help make dinner,* I said. Neither of us mentioned that he had numerous friends and relatives in the city, and money enough to rent a hotel for the night.

Over dinner with people we both knew, he told the guests that he had watched me years ago from a window on the staircase. I had danced about the kitchen in my birthday suit after the dinner guests had gone home and my second husband had gone to bed. He said I finished off their glasses of wine, ate the leftovers, tossed dishes into the sink, and leaped about the kitchen to music he couldn't hear. *There's a name for that. Peeping Tom,* I complained. If he intended to lessen my inhibitions with his story, he only frightened me into wondering how often I had entertained his renters and how much my body had changed over the years.

After the guests left, we sat in front of the fire, tossing logs onto the grate when the flame threatened to expire, choosing new music when the music died, seeming to have an endless stream of talk. I wasn't worried about bedtime because I had left other men at the guest-room door when they had visited from out of town. Flowers, chocolates, sweet words, and loneliness had not come between me and my fear of making yet another mistake.

The next morning, I could not remember what Noel and I had talked about. The wine bottle was empty, the guest bed untouched. Noel had disappeared from my bed and into an airplane headed for Montreal. I did not hear from him for two weeks. When he returned, he joined his friends in the pub after work. I learned many months later that he told his colleagues, *I think I'm in love.* But he did not tell me.

I planned to avoid him if he called, but when I heard his car drive up, I recognized my pleasure in Chance's tail; she wagged it like a pendulum on amphetamines. Noel bounded up the stairs with a bouquet of long-stemmed red roses. I tried to look stern, but my smile betrayed me. The dog squeezed between us as he handed me the flowers. He wore such a goofy smile that I invited him in to share the sweet lies that would soothe my pride. When he wasn't forthcoming, I tried to sound nonchalant: *Why didn't you call?* I asked. *I had a cold and I wanted to think,* he said. *In Montreal?* I said. *I have an old auntie and uncle there,* he explained. It was clear to me that this man needed a woman to teach him how to lie.

As new couples do, we cautiously shared our versions of days with others. After a few weeks, he let me know that he considered me unreasonable when I monopolized our conversations with details about the disorder of my second marriage. *Milton equated chaos with hell*, I told him. *Well, you're not there now*, he reminded me. Noel said he grew bored with having *three* of us over candlelight and wine, and that there were no answers to the past except to get on with the *now*. I agreed in theory but was remiss in reality, and that's when he came up with a compromise. I could argue with my phantoms until the clock struck noon. Then I had to stop and let the day be ours. Over time, he negotiated the hour of my selective pathos to an earlier and earlier one. By the end of the first year, I could seldom open my eyes in time to complain and, when I did, I could not wake him to listen. He insisted that *we* were the point. Otherwise he behaved like a rational man.

Life around our relationship changed, too. I was no longer subject to the slings and arrows of outrageous bias against divorced women. My colleagues saw me as saving face and growing content. Close friends no longer worried about my safety or tried to include me as the odd number for dinner, disappointed by my refusal to link up with their lonesome male acquaintants. Noel and I liked each other's friends and found ourselves surrounded by open doors. Best of all, I regained the anonymity and respect, however undeserved it might be, that people permit a committed woman. Our commuting relationship appealed to our independence, as well, giving us time to be solitary during the week. Each Friday one of us would take the ferry and the other would cook dinner. Chance spent the following summer being spoiled by my first in-laws while Noel and I wandered around Turkey, discovering each other in the noise of Istanbul, the meadows of Ephesus, and the sands of the Mediterranean.

Nothing stays the same. After two years, we set off an explosion and I was responsible for lighting the fuse. I took a summer's leave from Camosun College in Victoria, where I had worked for almost a decade, and accepted a job teaching at U.B.C. in Vancouver. I cycled to campus in the morning after Noel went off to his job, each of us doing work we enjoyed, each coming home to the person we wanted to see. We walked Chance along the trails of the neighboring forest that edges the campus, and we learned to do separate things while occupying the same room.

The neighbors laughed when, in a spontaneous act of charity, Noel gave his Buick to an old friend and bought a convertible to prove that he was not the conservative I had accused him of being. I was washing swallow droppings off the front steps in an effort to keep the cats from noticing the nest over the front alcove, when someone beeped. I turned but did not recognize either the dark green Mustang or the man in the straw hat. When he beeped again, I got annoyed. Just as my face grew hot with anger, I recognized the goofy grin behind the windshield.

During those two months, while European musicians rented my Victoria house for the city's six-week music festival and I lived in Noel's Vancouver home, we drove through the mountains around Vancouver, top down, sun shining, hanging onto our hats. Chance sat in the back on the new leather upholstery, her nose in the air and her short curls flattened by the wind. We hiked on the snow at Mount Baker, explored the Gulf Islands, and drove up to Whistler. Everything seemed new.

When the car was stolen six months later and dismantled near the border, we were grateful that we had been indulgent with ourselves and Chance, the dog Noel had initially relegated to the back porch. I wasn't surprised when he invited her into the car; I had caught them sitting together on his Persian rug, watching football and sharing popcorn. *She was a bit lonely,* he explained without being asked. The neighbors whispered to him that I was a hard worker when they saw me planting flowers on his deck. Jane Austen was right: no one wants to leave an unmarried man in his single state, especially people who suspect they might have been happier without wedding vows.

We both assumed we would regain our equilibrium when I returned to begin September with my students in Victoria. Perhaps the time had come to contemplate growing old with dignity. In our happiness we kept forgetting that we were no longer creeping into middle age: we had arrived. I was weeks from my fiftieth birthday. Permanent faculty positions were hard to come by, and I had left more than one to follow my second husband when he changed jobs. I would never again move on the whim of a man – especially one who had not yet asked me to. Instead, I had to relearn getting through the weekdays that interrupted our weekends, weekends that had once come before I was ready.

Noel cheered us up by buying tickets to San Francisco to celebrate my birthday. This trip was the beginning of my realization that I was growing tired of rushing away for weekends and hurrying back to the classroom. My only responsibility in getting to San Francisco was to take Chance to the kennel and catch an airplane for Vancouver. In late Friday afternoon traffic, with the dog in the back seat, my car's radiator blew up. The Honda had served me for thirteen faithful years and I had forgotten to return the favor by draining its antifreeze after four years of Okanagan winters. I flagged down a benevolent taxi driver who drove Chance to her kennel and me to my plane. When I gave him a large tip, he quarreled for less.

Noel and I were both returning to San Francisco after many years. In the early 1970s, he had been in California when he was working toward his Ph.D., and I had visited the city on my way to Mexico with my second husband in a camper van. The luxury hotel Noel had booked us into had no balcony or windows that opened onto the spectacular view. We were prisoners behind plate glass. When we stepped through the revolving doors, we felt guilty about the destitute people of all ages who begged for coins while we were being frivolous. The trolley cars picked up our spirits, but the once rustic wharf had become commercialized beyond our interest. When the ferry traffic poured into the streets of Sausalito, we experienced our biggest shock. The tiny artists' colony had become an expensive suburb with modern boutiques. I came away with a beautiful leather bag, but the joy of browsing and talking to artists in rough wooden shops was a delight of the past. These disappointments were eased considerably by the city's fabulous bookstores and restaurants, but we came home with reservations about the wonders of escaping for a three-day weekend in airports and air-conditioned hotels when we could have relaxed at home with popcorn, foreign movies, and longs walks.

Amid all this rushing back and forth, Noel solved our problem by deciding to quit his job, sell his house, and move to Victoria. I was paralyzed by the weight of responsibility and had to remind myself not to take seriously the promises of a man in love. He found a house with an acre of waterfront in Victoria and suggested I could move into it while he finished his job in Vancouver. In an uncharacteristic gesture of joy, he leapt into the air on a downtown street and clicked his heels together. I brought him back to earth by refusing to move with Chance away from the neighborhood where we were familiar and safe, and to live alone on the ocean-side. The house sold while we hesitated. We then agreed that he would sell his house and move into mine while we found a new house for both of us. Apprehensive and proud, we later talked of owning separate houses, in spite of the expense. We even searched for two shelters before we realized that our plural request to the realtor had changed into a singular one.

After six months, Noel moved into my house and we began our house hunting in earnest. Coming home after yet another futile search, I heard him sigh: *Oh all right. We'll renovate this house.* While my heart leapt for joy, he agreed to buy half my house and to renovate it into *our* new home with two phones, two studies, a new kitchen, bedroom, and sunroom – the illusion of independence combined with the joy of togetherness, a familiar place for Chance, and easy access to long ocean walks. Together we chopped carrots and baked scones in our new kitchen while Bruce Cockburn sang about *a great big love sweeping across the sky.*

I even resurrected an old dream to begin studies toward a Ph.D. I applied to the University of Victoria, for a leave from my teaching, and for considerable funding. I got all three, but I also got tired. As I pushed forward, my body began to push back, to argue with my ambitions, to demand rest. The newspaper suggested that a woman of fifty would be better to have plastic surgery than a Ph.D. I stepped up my exercise at the expense of my rest. Anything more serious than an abscessed tooth never crossed my mind. *Memento mori* was for those who were unhappy.

In April, between teaching my final college classes and invig-ilating my students' exams, I flew with Noel to Toronto for a family wedding at the King Edward Hotel. There I met his extended family: siblings, uncles, cousins, nieces, and nephews. No one in the immediate family had married outside their Jewish faith. No one had been divorced. When Noel's mother discovered that her bachelor son had given up his freedom to settle in with a divorced Gentile who had been married not once but twice and who did not seem intent on marrying again, she replied immediately: *Oy veh! Oy veh!* before she burst into a smile.

My introduction to Noel's family and the security they felt in their cloistered world caused me to ponder society's bias toward those who must endure not only divorce with all its immediate sorrow and emptiness, but also the connotations of the word *divorcée*. In the flawed reflection that the divorced woman acquires, the mirror of society dissolves her sense of place. Noel's family looked picture-perfect and seemed oblivious to despair. At dinner, I was seated beside his favorite auntie, a woman of ninety-two who lived in Montreal. She told me of her years in a concentration camp where she lost both her sister and her husband. I began to realize that joy comes from contrast as much as from success.

Noel's sister took a different tack upon meeting me than her mother or aunt had. She said hello, how *old* are you. I told her fifty-two. She returned later to repeat the question. I was reminded of my father's worry for my survival when I was single and momentarily disillusioned. In spite of my experience, he saw me as an innocent in a world of deceit. To Noel's mother, he would always be the recipient of her ineffectual worry, and to his sister he would always be baby brother. To me he was the most grown-up male I had ever encountered in close quarters.

When Noel flew back to Victoria and his office, I flew to Ottawa to visit a friend on sabbatical there. After the excitement of meeting Noel's family, I relaxed in the company of a woman who knew me well, someone I had shared sports and travels with in our years at the college together. Jenny and I wandered around the city, caught up on each other's news, played Scrabble, read, and made meals together. With her husband, we dined out at an Italian restaurant and went to the theater to see *Piaf.* I slept in their yellow guest room, and in its comforts I began – repeatedly, unaccountably, unstoppably – to cough.

Our world of dreams changed when, just before Christmas, my biopsy suggested lung cancer. Statistics forced us to ponder the idea that we might not grow old enough to stand the test of time. With the news, Noel began carrying our now aged Chance up and down the stairs. Her fifteen-year-old legs could no longer bend easily and neither of us could ask the vet to put her down. When I could not sleep, Noel strummed his guitar and sang songs in his off-key baritone voice. Lines from Leonard Cohen ring in my memory: *Dance me to your beauty/with a burning violin/Dance me through the panic/till I'm gathered safely in.*

When I was hospitalized, Noel got up before dawn to bring me breakfast, drive to his new job, return at noon to walk Chance, and go back to work before he ended his day by bringing me organic dinners to ward off the hospital food and taking the dog for her nightly hobble. We played Scrabble with the board resting on my thighs, perspiration dripping onto my wooden letters as I struggled with fever. I tried to think of seven-letter words that did not hint of death and yet counted for a lot. *Maturity* and *devotion* had one letter too many unless I could find words on the board to tie into.

Will you marry me? Noel asked, soon after he had brought me home from my last chemotherapy treatment and my first promising x-ray. I was sitting beside him in bed reading through drugstore glasses and wearing a flannelette nightie to keep me from post-surgery chill. *Maybe I will and maybe I won't,* I said, getting into the spirit. *Well, let me know if you decide,* he said, turning out his lamp. I finished the paragraph I was reading in Alice Munro and slipped my glasses down my nose to grin at him. In that moment of playfulness I caught the studied look in his eyes. *Maybe I will,* I said, as two decades of stress slipped from my bones and I joined him in the safety of our dreams.

I confess that I did not expect to marry again. In fact, I had lost all interest in marriage as a workable institution, at least for myself. My first and passionate ten-year marriage had disintegrated in the sorrow of our inability to have children, and my second, chaotic twelve-year marriage had begun with my next husband's lengthy pursuit of me and ended with his lengthy infidelity. I had had enough to do with *I do's.* To my ears, the operative part of the word *wedlock* was *lock.* Being someone's wife, I had reasoned, was not the only way of *being,* and I had set out to prove that I could make my own way.

But a problem lurked in the shadow of my upbringing. As I've said, I am the daughter of a man who had loved not only my mother but also my sisters, our dog, our canary, my maternal grandmother, and me. In a phrase, he was *a family man.* And try as I might I could never quite shake off the notion that a man of his moral stature, devotion, and humor was strolling down the beach with his dog or curled up with his books and music or penciling out renovations, waiting for me to rescue him from life's harsh disappointments.

After Noel and I agreed to marry, I began to wake with a sense of well-being that I had forgotten in the years preceding my diagnosis. He asked me what I was dreaming about that made me smile in my sleep. When he came home late from a meeting one evening, he discovered me deep in the Land of Nod with something clutched in my hands and propped on my chest under the quilt. When he turned back the covers, he found a cup full of milky Ovaltine without a drop spilled. More surprising was that the cup was propped on the untouchable – my scar. Bedtime became my favorite time as I let go of my need to keep watch over myself and relaxed into knowing that I would not awaken before dawn speckled the room. I would not have described myself as happy. It would have been too much temptation for the gods.

In the following weeks I tried to regain my senses but I kept slipping into the languor of being at home in my own skin. A mother pushing her baby in a grocery cart as I rummaged among the organic vegetables prompted me to look again rather than to look away. I found everyone smiling at me, and I realized they were responding to my smile. I began mentioning my up-coming nuptials to friends, expecting them to say, *Why bother?* or *Haven't you learned anything yet?* Instead they asked to be included in the celebration, to have a reason to dust off spring hats and bring dress-up clothes out of their closets, to buy film and drink wine in the afternoon. Their middle-aged enthusiasm seemed to derive from the idea that we had finally come to our senses. Cancer or no, divorced or not, something sweet was trying to be born.

Just as suddenly as I had become happy, I grew edgy. All this good will frightened me. For the better part of two weeks, I expected our house to collapse in an earthquake or be flooded by early spring rains. I watched for a car to turn unexpectedly into my lane or a pervert to jump out from behind a tree. I imagined a wayward branch poking my eyeball. My fears ended on the back deck one sunny morning with a voice from my past: *You were always a sweet thing, but so hard to help,* my mother whispered. I had not realized before that she had been trying to coax me to trust in love, to let go of the myth that fear would protect me.

Why, I wonder, does our world revolve around *love?* The emotion it fuels differs so much from the *knowing* of something. It allowed me to turn away from the past and peek into the future. If I had to think of a moment that I recognized love's return, I would say it came when a stronger hand than my own reached across the bed and rested on the spot that marked the heart of my cancer, a place that had been bruised by my second husband's fist. With Noel's touch, I saw my breast as the home of a wound that needed kindness to heal.

But the timing of his proposal bewildered me. After all, surgery had corrugated a narrow strip of skin between my breasts, and the chemotherapy and radiation treatments had played Delilah to my Samson, enticing me forward but lessening my strength. I reminded him that I could no longer even breathe with the same clarity as before. *Who knows what's happened to my kidneys and liver?* We had lived apart and together in relative harmony for five years. Now, in our sixth year, why had we arranged for two trumpeters to herald our wedding celebration as a symbol of great joy? Perhaps I wondered what his family with its three doctors would think of his marrying a woman who may not be around to bury the dead, as Jung suggested a woman should do. Seeking assurance, I mustered up courage to ask what had inspired him to say those four words. After all, he had avoided the question for all of his adult life. *Four more,* he answered with a ridiculous grin – *You're still in there.*

We began our wedding plans with the notion of organizing a day that would be festive for family and friends. The first step was to find someone to marry us. In our case this was more complicated than it is for many people. We did not wish to repeat anything from our pasts or to settle for an impersonal ceremony at City Hall. Noel had always opted for common-law relationships; I had married first in my late teens in a church wedding with a formal reception in a banquet hall on the Saskatchewan prairies, and the second time in a garden with champagne and lamb-on-a-spit in Vancouver's Kitsilano. Noel and I chose to marry under an enormous willow tree in the gardens that slope to the sea on the grounds of a heritage Tudor building called the Oak Bay Beach Hotel. It sits on a stretch of ocean facing Mount Baker with its mighty glacier, a mountain on which Noel had exposed the foolishness of love by diving into a glacial lake to prove on the instant that he too could swim in freezing waters, as I had once done.

Our cultural backgrounds created another difference. I had been christened an Anglican and raised a Presbyterian in the United Church, gone to its summer camp as a child, sung in its choir as a teen-ager, and taught Sunday school as a young adult. Noel had been born into the Jewish culture and had attended the synagogue as a boy, had his ritual circumcision there as an infant and his bar mitzvah when he entered his teens. A Jewish friend, who had once married a gentile woman and was about to marry another, suggested that the Unitarian Church might be the place to start.

In acknowledgment of our pasts, we also arranged to have two wedding songs, a Hebrew song sung *a cappella* in a haunting minor key by a young singer with the sweetest voice on earth and a love song by Stephen Sondheim called "Not a Day Goes By." We also decided to have our parents' wedding pictures beside our enormous chocolate cake to accompany Noel's mother, our only living parent. It would later make us laugh to look at them standing in the slimness of their photographs amid the bulbous sugared fruit on its bed of deep chocolate. Finally, I took my first step toward the marriage ceremony by calling Reverend Vann Knight, whose Unitarian Church sits on the peninsula of West Saanich with its horses and lambs, cows and ostriches that dot the farmlands from Victoria to the ferry docks.

When the minister answered the phone, I described our different pasts and asked if he could officiate at the service. His answer delighted me: *You all come to the right place*, he said in a southern drawl. *I have to have this voice,* I thought. After a brief conversation, I realized that nothing in his accent or his choice of words suggested either old-world droning or new-age navel-gazing. On our way to meet Reverend Knight, I brought up a subject Noel and I usually avoided. *Do you have to tell him you're an atheist?* I asked in the sweetest voice I could muster. Noel considered the request in silence, then answered in true-to-male fashion: *Don't you worry about it.* In the minister's study in a rambling heritage house, Reverend Knight asked me about my religious past and then shared stories of his own. In this comfortable atmosphere, he turned to Noel. *I consider myself an atheist*, my betrothed began. Soon the two men had forgotten the future bride as they talked congenially about philosophy, history, and family origins.

When we got down to the mechanics of the ceremony, the minister offered three suggestions that would allow our separate cultures to flow together. One was the Jewish custom of holding a canopy over the marrying couple, the second was the ritual of candles, and the third was the glass-breaking ceremony. We declined the first in favor of nature's canopy of sky and trees, but agreed to the candles and the glass-breaking. I expressed my concern that

Noel and I would have to take special care not to allow *my* candle to blow out in the breeze. I explained that everyone including the groom would fear the dying of the light represented an end to my remission, a darkness come before the dawn of marriage. *We have to keep my candle lit,* I said with more force than I had intended. That's when Reverend Knight told us that he too had been divorced and that his new wife had also endured a startling cancer. We left with the sense that we were an odd trio of kindred spirits and that Noel and I had chosen well.

We also left with the project of searching out three candle holders, each with a hurricane glass, and of finding a wine glass for our memorable day. We found the candlesticks by accident one day when we passed an art shop. The hand-blown stems differ slightly from each other, and on top of each are four copper claws that hold up both the candle and its tall and frosted hurricane glass that protects the flame against a breeze. We bought these saffron candle holders to stand on either side of another, larger, carved wooden candle holder with its transparent wind glass. These three works of art seemed perfect for our May wedding.

In the ritual of candles, the matching pair represents the *chi* or life forces of the bride and groom, each with its own beauties and flaws. The more solid central candle represents marriage, as the mating pair come together. During the ceremony, each partner lights his or her candle and then together they light the central one with their separate flames. Once lit, the three candles symbolize a combined illumination, spreading a greater light and warmth than one could do alone. As with life, all three candles will eventually falter, but together their temporary flames spread a glorious light before their final flicker.

The tradition of breaking glass involves the couple's sharing sweet wine from a single goblet. The groom wraps the empty glass in a towel and stomps on it. Fleetingly I objected to being barred from the stomping process, but considered my delicate wedding shoes and let the rule of King Kong hold sway. The shattering of glass represents the broken dreams a couple must endure if their marriage is to succeed, and the number of shards signifies the sweet years they will share. Our vessel turned out to be sitting behind the leaded glass of our china cabinet. It had once been part of a gold-rimmed pair I had bought years before, but it now sat alone, beautiful and unused, a keepsake needing a new role.

On the day we set off to buy dessert wine to fill this glass, and dry wines for our pre-nuptial dinner, Noel and I took the Malahat Highway north of Victoria to the village of Cobble Hill. Here Gordano and Marilyn, an Italian man and his English wife, entertain guests and live with their children on the edge of their organic vineyard. Noel and I were invited to join another couple at a long dining-room table in front of a stone fireplace to sample the wines. Although we tend, since my illness, to restrict our alcohol to weekend dinners or social gatherings, we sipped various dessert wines before we chose one. La Rocca, the fortress, whose sweet taste came from an exquisite bottle in the shape of a dinner bell, had the effect of making its recipient feel safe from all the problems that afflict mankind. With one decision made, we went on to try various dinner wines until we chose Millefiori, a thousand flowers, for the pre-nuptial gathering. By the time we'd slurred out our choice and ordered four cases, we were certain our union had been blessed by the gods and that the strangers around the table were our lasting friends. After lurching forward in our car and giggling at something neither of us can now recall, we pulled off the road and waited for sobriety to revisit us.

And so it came to be that I woke on the morning of May 11, 1996, to dress for my wedding day. We had sent invitations that had pictures of ourselves at age four, Noel riding a tricycle with the same mischievous smile he would later wear as he drove a car, and I sitting on my parents' couch looking as though I hoped I was pleasing someone. I stepped into my bathroom with my hairdresser and came out with calla lilies peeking from the folds of my upswept hair. My stepdaughter from my second marriage, Camille, helped me climb into the dress that a clever designer had made to hug my best spots and hide my worst. It draped slim and long to the floor in the shimmering color of sun on prairie wheat. My matron of honor, Jenny, and my bridesmaid, Trudy, arrived to dress in their silky suits of silvery blue and antique rose. Everyone contrived to keep hidden from me for tradition's sake the man I had been sleeping with for almost six years.

From my ears dangled two ribbons of *old* gold with a diamond hanging from the bottom of each. The right earring had been made from the gold of my first wedding band in combination with the melted gold of my first husband's ring. This diamond was the one he had given me when I was nineteen. The matching left earring was made from the gold of my second wedding band; I had bought a diamond to match the first one. Noel's and my *new* rings were made by the same artist – simple bands, differing only in the diamond that Noel had insisted I have and that I had asked to be deeply buried in the gold so I could wear the ring for hiking as easily as for dining out. Our hands had been hard to fit, my finger slightly smaller than the smallest band on the metal measuring rings and his slightly larger than the biggest one. We had found our match in simplicity, mine eventually fitting snug inside his on the night table while we slept.

While Jenny and Trudy talked with my younger brother-in-law, Ken, I caught myself in a moment of rising sadness. Together in my kitchen were three people who had been flawless supporters during my illness, and yet something was missing. I realized the source of my hollow feeling: What was a wedding without my family? Before I could contemplate an answer, I felt their presence upon me, warming my blood, easing my soul. My elder sister would have remembered her own youthful wedding when she was dressed in white silk and lace. I thought of my younger sister's face and hoped she had remembered the significance of the day even though she had chosen not to join us. I knew my mother would think I looked beautiful in long lace sleeves that reached to my fingers and matched the design of her own silk gown, a wedding dress she had made in her family farmhouse sixty years before and that now hung in my closet. I imagined her smile as I turned to show her the covered buttons that reached from my neck to my tailbone. I smiled too as I thought of how I had managed to alter by two decades my mother's suggestion that *a woman's life begins at thirty.* Time had replaced one bride with another, but the underlying drift of hope remained. I knew too that my father's spirit would rest easy in his unwavering definition of love: *It means finding joy in the other person's joy and refusing to harbor bad times.* My family was all around me, its sun sparkling as dew on the morning grass.

I was, as well, keeping a promise I had intended to make years before over my parents' shared grave. I had gone to the cemetery to pledge that I would show some prairie stamina and let go of the wounds from my second marriage. Instead I had sunk onto my knees and sobbed into the grass of Sunnyside Lawn, my hands on its newly laid stone: *I'm doing the best I know how.* The past and the present, my parents' love and Noel's, had given me strength to move forward.

In the calm of the moment, I remembered the one promise I had left unfulfilled. I had not yet prepared my wedding vows to surprise Noel as he said he had done days before. No words seemed adequate. Ken called into my reverie: *Do you want me to hold the hand that you put through my arm?* I was surprised and grateful. *Yes. Please. Hang onto me until you give me away.* Ken teased, *Can someone just give you away?* We had to look away to keep our emotions intact. Ken, Jenny, and Trudy climbed into the waiting white Daimler with me as two elderly grannies in the neighborhood waved us off with flowers.

Voices overflowed the lobby of the hotel. Noel and I had agreed to marry in the large hall that overlooked the water and the mountain if wind and dampness made the stone stairs too slippery for the elderly to descend to the garden. The tiger lilies on the grand piano seemed to open to the music of the pianist, and the trumpeters waited between their jazz duets and their "Trumpeter's Wedding March" as I began down the polished wooden stairs. A crowd of familiar faces ranging from a seven-month-old baby to Noel's eighty-nine-year-old mother hushed as the trumpeters raised their horns.

As in a slow dream, Ken and I moved into the sound of the trumpets. Down the makeshift aisle, I passed old friends from Vancouver and my graduate days at U.B.C., and colleagues and friends from Victoria. My widowed brother-in-law and a niece and a nephew from my elder and younger sisters' families stood beside a cluster of Noel's extended family. Our six-year-old godchild watched her father standing with Noel. My neighbors stood next to my first mother-in-law, who had known me since I was fifteen. The guests reached into all the pockets of our past and present. The years of my life had come together to carry us into a realm of mutual hope.

But some intuitive fear stirred in me. The cake had arrived before the guests had gathered and a cornucopia of food and wine was waiting. Noel's sister, a willowy blonde with a love of gatherings and a sense of humor, had agreed to toast the groom. One of my dearest colleagues, a man with a love for poetry, had agreed to give the toast to the bride. I knew he would speak with an eloquence that would soothe ears and lift spirits, as he did with his students. Although we had never spoken of it, I also knew that he would find lines from Yeats, and the afternoon proved my prophecy: *Think where a man's glory will begin and end, / And say my glory is that you're my friend.*

But my apprehension had almost reached a breaking point by the time I neared the altar (or in this case, the fireplace). Noel watched me with shy calmness as I approached him, his brother, his friend of thirty years, and Reverend Knight. Noel wore a yellow silk tie with blue flowers to match his dark blue suit. The white velvet faces of big Casablanca lilies looked up from their pot on the stone floor beside the fireplace. When I saw Jenny and Trudy turn to watch me, I realized that my moment of truth had arrived and that my dress hem was quivering. Noel's eyes spoke of a private joy when I reached him, and I steadied myself by looking into his face.

He kept his eyes on me, and without faltering in words or gaze, he gave his long and passionate vows about looking after me and sharing in my life *until we walk off into the sunset that sets over the water at the end of our street.* I could hear guests blowing their noses before a silence followed, which I was supposed to fill. I knew then why I had gone unprepared. I no longer wanted to make up vows I couldn't keep without the luck of the gods and the goodness of my partner. Instead I wanted to respond to someone else's plan, someone I could trust to be strong when I was not. I was tired of trying and I wanted simply to be me, and so I promised *to help to make these dreams come true for us and to obey him* – I heard mutterings from feminist friends who had to be told later that I had qualified my promise of obedience by admitting what I could not do alone – take care of my health. At this point Reverend Knight said it was time for the lighting of candles.

With combined purpose, we lit our separate candles that stood on a small table nearby. Looking into each other's eyes, we leaned forward to light from these the larger one. Noel's candle hit the table with an audible thud, snuffing out the light that represented his half of the bargain. More than a hundred guests seemed to breathe in at once as we looked across at the floundering culprit that rolled down the tablecloth like a log set dangerously free from a log jam. Noel swept up the delinquent candle as I pondered the benefits of the candle glue I had nonchalantly refused as unpoetic. *Light it from mine*, I whispered, finding at last my missing vow. And that was the moment our wedding came to life. Noel jammed his candle into the holder, leaned it into mine, and we kept steady to each other's light as we joined our *chi* in the central flame.

Did you hear that, folks? the minister cried out. *Did you hear? Light it from mine,* he repeated in his glorious accent, and he was off and running with a straight-from-the-heart speech that left cynics and idealists, young and old, married and single guests blowing their noses and dabbing their eyes. At the moment of crisis, the minister's spontaneity had joined us as *helpmeets,* just as the Old Testament of our two religions suggests to be the truth of marriage.

His blessings followed the prayer: *In this hour, rich with meaning and hope and promise, we pray that the spirit of trust, understanding, and love may be with you now and forever.*

Noel and I shared our heady wine by linking arms and sipping in turn from the gold-rimmed glass before he smashed it to smithereens in one fell stomp. Reverend Knight declared us husband and wife and invited us to greet each other with a kiss. As Noel's lips touched mine, the trumpeters raised their brass flowers toward the heavens. I took his hand, and together we moved into the celebration. The music of the recessional swept out into the garden, reaching across the ocean and toward the snow-capped mountain.

❦ 9 ❦

A Parable of
Fireflies

Having been swallowed into the belly of cancer and then fished out by hope, I found myself in my second year of remission, once again a woman in the midst of her life. After the last wedding guests had kissed us good-bye, Noel and I escaped to Sooke Harbour House. On the way we passed the wooden chapel where Kathleen's friends had last gathered to remember her. I squeezed Noel's hand.

At the hotel, he lifted me over the threshold of our room and we sank into opposite ends of a Jacuzzi tub. Noel bent his long legs to make room for my short ones, and together we drank mineral water and looked out on waves and sky. When dusk began to fall and we had grown calm enough to feel hungry again, we found warm housecoats in the closet and fruit, smoked salmon, and champagne outside our door. With no sound other than a crackling fire, we were drawn into the tenderness of the night.

At home, I began packing for our honeymoon flight to Italy while Noel prepared for his absence from work. Our month-long trip was an offshoot of a postponed holiday. We had rented a villa in Tuscany for the summer of 1994, but Noel's move to Victoria, our renovations, and my cough had depleted our appetite for change. Feeling penny-pinched and disoriented, we pushed our plan forward to the next summer and sat down on our new deck. In the summer of 1995, after my cancer treatments, we chose to ferry to an island retreat five hours from home where eating and sailing were our only responsibilities. In the company of gentle strangers, I learned to see my disease with some objectivity, and to begin writing in private about the fears and blessings that accompany its visit.

I tried to convince myself that I was not much different from those without cancer, that each life is a matter of moments that blossom into memorable times or shrivel into forgettable ones. But when we finally bought our tickets to Rome, I did not think about being there as I had always done on previous trips; I thought about getting there. Elena had suggested that I fly with an oxygen tank and my radiation oncologist had arranged the paperwork. I was no longer an innocent, taking life for granted. The scourge of radiation and the poison of chemotherapy had done a job on my spirit as well as my body, and remission was accompanied by a keen sense of vulnerability. I speculated that a stray cancer cell could turn my bravado into foolishness, that a sore arm could turn an ache into bone cancer, that a toothache might expose a brain metastasis, that a bloated stomach could be the first signs of a malignant liver.

To reach Rome I had to overcome my daunting apprehension. This fear of flying had little in common with Erica Jong's. Noel and I could have our erotic fling *after* touching ground in Italy. My fear had to do with being enclosed in the narrow confines of a metal tube in air that was on recycle. As we waited for the flight to Toronto and its connecting flight to Rome, I had an ominous thought. In April 1994, after a wedding in Toronto, this very flight in reverse had marked the beginning of my respiratory problem – a cold, a cough, and an all-consuming exhaustion.

Now, two years later, on the plane to Rome, a flight attendant lugged my oxygen tank down the aisle. *Can you manage?* she asked. *That's why I brought a man,* I said, surprised by the tank's size and grateful for Noel's broad shoulders and long arms. My upper body had been bereft of strenuous exercise since surgery and radiation. *Put your thumb over the air hole and watch for the balloon to inflate,* the attendant cautioned. Noel put the tank under my feet and slithered down to assemble the parts. Muttering to himself, his head pressed against my calf, he attached the tube and fidgeted with the valve to free oxygen to move from tank to tube to mask to me. *Is it happening?* he asked. I stuck my thumb over the opening to my mask and watched the test balloon inflate. We both grinned, and I adjusted the mask over my face while other passengers watched. *It looks ridiculous,* I whispered. *Who cares?* he said. *Just keep breathing.* In a short time I had forgotten that my reading glasses were propped up by the plastic mask. I remembered when I jabbed the mask with a forkful of lunch.

Our rented villa in Tuscany was planned as the safety net where I would learn that, with precautions, I could travel again. When Noel persuaded me we would rent a car in Rome to assure easy access to the villa or to medical help, I felt as though I had lapsed from an adventurer into a tourist. En route to Italy, though, I began to escape for long moments from the nagging fear of cancer's return. Perhaps I simply exchanged it for other fears. *What other fears?* Noel asked as we hobbled off the plane, sleep deprived and stiff. *It's just an inexplicable inner gasp,* I explained. Since becoming sick, I had grown afraid of things I had never contemplated before, such as accidents and earthquakes. Noel put his arm around my shoulder and we rode the moving aisle to the car rental depot in the airport.

On the highway, we glimpsed comforting orange phone boxes

with S.O.S. signs. As a Maserati flew past us, I heard Noel complain to our lime-green Lancia as he pressed the accelerator to the floor. Somewhere in the blur we swerved toward a secondary road, but to get off the autostrada we had to pay. We had no idea how to work the toll gate or communicate our problem to the attendant, who remained behind a glass wall waiting for a magic card that we did not have. Finally, as the line-up behind us grew with our exasperation, the attendant fiddled with his computer and the gate lifted to free us from the first leg of our journey. *Pretty good trick,* I teased. Embarrassed, Noel drove in silence toward a lesser road.

Lesser has nothing to do with speed. It simply means two lanes of maniacal drivers instead of four. In front of us, a sultry beauty on a moped weaved through the traffic. As we caught up with her, she tilted into the passing lane to slip between the truck in front of her and an oncoming car. Italians drive like skiers on a slalom course, missing obstacles by a sparrow's wing. On our third try, we too managed to pass the truck, and I was able again to admire the free-spirited loveliness of the woman, her long hair blowing and her mustard-colored skirt flapping behind her. When we passed her, my eye was drawn from her high-heeled shoes and exposed thighs to her hands. One gripped the accelerator; the other raised and lowered a cigarette.

Eventually we turned off our motor at a resort on a large lake. In early evening we bought wine, bread, olives, and cheese to eat on the lake shore. Three mallards entertained us by unabashedly trying to copulate with a lone female who was doing her best to get on with dinner. Apparently divorce was not standard practice in the duck world; a female simply had to put up with her life's accumulation of mistaken hopes. I shared my remaining bread crumbs with her.

At dawn from our balcony we could see mist clinging to the lake. Fishermen moved into the still water; birds skimmed through the haze. We drove to the medieval city of Sutri, where we got our morning exercise and began breaking the rules of diet for cancer survivors. The walking was robust in the angular climbs to unexpected dead ends that once fooled the enemy and now fool the tourist. But all paths eventually lead to the central piazza, where we found an outdoor table. Our *caffè latte* combined two forbidden items – a stimulant and a dairy product. Oh, the tangled web we weave.

Our illusions about knowing enough of the language to order meals with ease soon dissolved. Sometimes we had happy accidents, like our pasta with garlic sauce so powerful it spiced up our kisses for the remainder of the day. This bulb holds an Olympic place in the realm of health foods that help the immune system. Our new perception made appealing the former unpleasantness of garlic breath.

As a supposedly terminal cancer patient, I had once wondered at the sense of buying new clothes. Now I idled at the shop windows in every village. Noel, who considers himself more sensible about finances, widened his eyes when I said, *Everything seems ridiculously cheap once you lop off those three extra zeros.* Lorna Crozier's "Poem about Nothing" explores the importance of *zero,* which is supposed to signify *nothing* and yet can enfold considerable meaning, especially when it slithers between numbers. *Zero worms its way/between one and one/and changes everything.* Just like cancer.

Out the windshield of our Lancia, red poppies matted the roadside between vineyards and wheat fields. Threshing had begun, and tidy bales spotted the Tuscan landscape like children's toys. In late afternoon, we entered the valley that surrounds Cortona, an ancient Etruscan town close to our villa. Noel passed the same crumbling church dome from three different angles – *Are you looking at the right map?* he asked, unimpressed by my navigational skills – and with the sun in our faces, we finally found a juncture that seemed rather like the one we were looking for. Passing a private property sign, we drove up to the house. Before us stood a small and unloved stone dwelling in an overgrown yard. Two rusty cars sat in the shade.

When Noel knocked on the door, no one answered. I wandered through the chaos of the yard but there was no sign of life or of the second cottage that was supposed to house us. *What do you think?* he asked. I thought of poisonous vipers slithering through the long grass and scorpions lurking in the shade of stone. Weariness caused a plug of fear to expand in my throat. I remembered reading that heat can spell trouble for the respiratory system. *Let's get out of here*, I said.

Our error was apparent once we found the right turnoff. A trimmed grass road with parallel tracks led us past two blond horses in a corral bordered by grape vines. The animals reminded me of a day in my girlhood when my father had surprised me by raising his voice in response to my hammering a picture of Roy Rogers and Trigger onto my bedroom wall. He was not angry about the objects of my infatuation, but about the large spikes I had driven into the four corners of my tiny picture. In Italy, away from customary surroundings, I often had flashes on the distant past. I realized with contentment that I had finally begun to think further back than my chemotherapy and radiation treatments.

Cool air rushed through our open windows and carried with it the duet of birds and creek. When the road opened into the sun, we saw three stone buildings surrounded by an enormous lawn edged with rose bushes. At one end, large pottery urns with red geraniums stood in front of a background of chestnut and oak trees. Our hosts, Sharon and Dan, had come out to welcome us. Beside them, a beautiful eighteenth-century cottage, in bygone days the miller's home, waited for us. Noel and I looked at each other, hearts flush, not daring to speak.

Sharon had put fresh poppies and carnations on the long narrow dining-room table, which sat on a burnished terra-cotta floor. A thick whitewashed wall separated this room from the kitchen, three steps down. It too had a fireplace, as well as a modern gas stove, and a long rough-hewn table with a bowl of apples, grapes, strawberries, basil, rosemary, sage, and thyme. The cupboards and walls held all the utensils and dishes for a gourmet cook. *You'll be in paradise*, I said, reminding Noel that he had promised during a moment of madness to do the cooking on our honeymoon in return for my having made our wedding invitations. Opening shuttered windows, I leaned out between billowing drapes and watched two white butterflies unite into one before cartwheeling into the trees.

Our days soon took on a lazy rhythm. Two or three times a week, I swished clothes around in the small upstairs bath and then called Noel to help me wring them into a damp pile. Outside, I kicked off my shoes and took our bucket of freshly washed clothes to the drying lines. Alone in the world, I rested my eyes on the orchard or let them sweep across the lawn below or into the distant countryside. I listened to the birds sing as the sun warmed my arms and the dry grass brushed my feet. It was nature's opera house, with its baritone doves, soprano cuckoos, and the liquid mezzo trill of woodlarks. When I saw the white and brown flash of the hoopoes, I was reminded of my mother pointing out robin nests to me while she stretched the family's sheets across the line to dry in the prairie breeze.

Around noon, I returned the pegs to their basket, folded the clothes, and stacked them on the dry grass. I breathed in the essence of warm wind in the fiber, and it soothed my recovering lungs, medicine dressed in the silken breeze of Tuscany. With each breath, I felt a connectedness to womankind from centuries past. For generations women had come from all around to wash their laundry under the small waterfall nearby and then offer it up to the sun. No woman who has participated in the rhythm of life is entirely forgotten; she leaves her mark on the heart's knowing, the subconscious spring that quenches our need to belong.

During our honeymoon, I realized why Southern European men have a reputation for being great lovers. In North America, many middle-aged men spend their workweek competing against the clock and following their stocks, only going to bed in the day if they take a mistress. In contrast, a Tuscan man luxuriates at home during a three-hour daily siesta, succumbing to the pleasures of food, wine, and slumber. Any negative emotions that may have plagued him earlier in the day have been assuaged at the wheel of his car, thumb on the horn and foot on the accelerator. Driving in Italy is a team sport, an encounter group. Once I asked Noel why he was beeping his horn when I couldn't see a car nearby. He said he was just practicing. I understood why Italians have a reputation for living long and abundant lives. After the midday luxury of Italian food and wine, Noel and I napped in the refreshing cool of our stone-walled bedroom. It was hard to keep *Eros* at bay under the great fluffy duvet and fresh sheets that our hosts had bought to welcome us, their first honeymoon guests. Great lovers may simply be well-fed and rested people tucked safely away from phones and computers.

On the days when our hosts were busy gardening, or had left

for town to buy groceries or wine, we threw off our clothes and ran a hot bath in the bedroom's small ensuite. We bathed one at a time because the tiny bath was shaped like a bench, and even then Noel's knees touched his chin. While I bathed, he stacked glasses and wine on a tray to bring to the bathroom, where he sat on the closed toilet to talk to me, warm wind from the open window on his back. It was always cool within the stone walls, making an afternoon rest a luxurious escape from one kind of heat into another. Afterward, I sneaked away while Noel slept. I tiptoed naked onto the upper lawn, where I could dance out my joy at being alive.

One morning, we decided to climb the back roads to Cortona. The day had begun to heat up as I looked through my small wardrobe for something that would allow the breeze to touch my skin. I unfolded a white cotton dress with its scooped neckline that I saved for travel. Glimpsing my scar in the mirror, I struggled to keep back tears. Unless I wore a T-shirt underneath the dress, my scar would show. I felt I had grown so much older on the outside than I was inside, although my lung specialists might have argued the point. And I remembered when I was nine years old, and my grandmother at sixty-nine had reflected aloud on this sentiment after burying my grandfather. I had caught the hurt look on her face when I asked if she had been pretty back then. I didn't understand what she meant when she cocked her chin and said, *I had it when I needed it.*

My lung surgery was a miracle of healing down to a point just above my breasts, where a knot had been tied over one of the staples that held my sternum together. An empty feeling came over me, as always without warning; it happens when I am doing something I have done often, but not since my surgery. Putting on my favorite summer dress was such an act, and it made me question why I bothered to travel, or to hope, or even to get out of bed. In spite of my philosophy of putting one foot in front of the other, to keep moving, I suddenly wanted to sink under the tiles and hide.

So much of my own small share of female beauty had resided in my breasts. If that pride had come before the usual age-induced fall, perhaps I would have found it as easy to accept as I have my reading glasses. But my anguish was compounded by guilt. I thought of the seven friends who had bravely endured surgery for breast cancer: three had lumpectomies, one had lost her left breast, a young mother had lost both breasts, and two had lost their lives. I thought too of my hostess's neighbor, who had gone to visit her children in the United States and come home without a breast. I would tell others that my scar was small potatoes and expect them to laugh at the double entendre.

The angry, asymmetrical tack of red flesh told me that no amount of exercise, no healthy diet, no loving hand could bring back the idea that in time the flesh repairs itself entirely. The scar seemed to hold in its small red fist an argument against my ever feeling free again. I relived the day when, after my shower, I had toweled off the mist on my mirror and for the first time looked directly at the results of the surgeon's blade. It took my breath away to glimpse the red line that ran from clavicle to solar plexus. I had to return to the same task morning after morning before I could finally say, *This is me now,* and realize I was lucky to be in a warm bathroom with Noel's towel hung next to mine.

As I fretted over my white dress, Noel caught me unaware. His eyes spoke of an understanding that made me want to hide in the woods for a good sulk. He sat on the edge of the bed and talked about a trip he had taken to Cuba years before with a girlfriend.

On the first morning, he had dived into the ocean feeling virile and young. When the salty waves washed over him, the blond hair he brushed back over his bald spot had plastered itself over his ears. He realized at that moment the meaning of self-acceptance. *I knew I was going to keep losing hair from here on in, that I wouldn't see a full head of hair in the mirror again.* He shrugged. His boyhood pride in his blond hair had become, in an instant, a memory. *I decided to lengthen my forehead by shortening my hair.* I stroked his cheek and leaned my head on his. *The rest of your hair's not even blond anymore,* I said, and we laughed.

I patted suntan lotion onto my scar, no longer sure whether it hurt or whether I simply imagined the pain, as a dog will do years after a wound has healed. I shut my eyes and ran my fingers over the groove, deciding that it felt more foreign than painful. Without looking in the mirror, I slipped into my dress and sandals. Outside Noel waited for me, and I tucked my hand into his as we walked along gravel tracks, through trees, and over a wooden bridge. Climbing to the city, I did my interpretation of J.J.Cale's *If you don't like my peaches, don't shake upon my tree.* Noel assured me he liked my peaches just as they were.

In Cortona we discovered a museum that houses treasures from Etruscan tombs, triptychs of saints from the Middle Ages, and paintings from the Renaissance to the twentieth century. My favorites were a small bronze Janus and an Etruscan chandelier as big as the circle of my arms, its many candle holders separated by faces carved in stone. At closing time, I expressed disappointment to the female official who was locking the doors, showing her a copy in the guide book of a painting I'd been unable to find. The woman gave me an enormous smile and took me back inside to a small room I had passed by. I showed her that in the museum's brochure the baby nursed from the mother's left breast but in the painting it nestled at her right. We laughed and spoke to each other in words that neither could translate except in the common language of a woman's heart. Her eyes never once strayed down to my scar.

Next we climbed to the top of the Medici fortress that allowed us to see over the city and down the valley; then we cooled off in a nearby cathedral. This church is famous for its glass coffin that holds the body of Santa Margherita. Her small form looks like a withered and discolored doll. These tanned-leather remains reminded me of my mortality, and I was again a cancer patient in remission. I slouched down on a pew and thought about how long it would be before I could talk with Elena or have a therapeutic massage or know that the clinic was just minutes away. A wizened priest in his long brown robe jostled me from my thoughts by expressing his considerable disgust that I had propped my bare feet on the kneeling bench. As my face grew hot and I tried to apologize, Noel interrupted. *Time to leave,* he said, ushering me out. We could hear the ancient celibate harassing someone else as the heavy doors closed behind us.

In the narrow Cortona street we sat drinking wine and eating pizza, too tired to talk. A black hearse passed by so close to our chairs that we could see individual petals on the bouquets decorating its top and sides. Mourners passed our table one by one, looking out their car windows, and I was reminded by their swollen eyes and wet cheeks that the privacy of our Canadian rituals is not common everywhere. Grief expresses the value of the lost person, and to an Italian it must be shared to complete the family's sense of closure. The hearse brought to mind the novels of Nino Ricci – *Lives of the Saints* and *In a Glass House* – in which he writes about suffocating in the physical and emotional density of Italian life and growing invisible in the vastness and restraint of Canada.

As the afternoon waned, we wandered down to the tenth-century stone church at the turnoff to our villa. After pulling open the heavy wooden doors, we rested a moment within its ancient walls. Except for fresh flowers on the altar, there was no sign that anyone had been around to light the candles. The late sun transformed the church windows, and I felt joined to the lives that had begun and ended here over years of christenings and funerals, joy and mourning. I recalled photos of myself and my sisters in our christening gowns; I shuddered at the memory of family funerals. *Are you cold?* Noel asked. *No,* I said, *just thinking about the things that take place in churches everywhere.* He smiled: *Like weddings?*

When we walked up the path to the villa, my dress was damp and wrinkled. I stopped in to tell Sharon that I had taken up scooped necklines with gay abandon. She gestured for me to hush. *Can you hear the dove cooing?* she asked in a lullaby voice, pointing to the nearby wood. It spoke of something haunting and ageless. After darkness had fallen and Noel and I had bathed and settled into our books, Sharon called through the window for us to look outside. *Hurry up!* Noel urged, standing in the open doorway. The nearby bushes were alight with hundreds and hundreds of fireflies. I imagined they were celebrating the luck of being born in the Tuscan countryside as they attracted their mates for the age-old dance. Finite time, infinite beauty – they twinkled from the edge of darkness, glittering confetti, diamonds in the night.

I would wash my dress to wear again tomorrow.

That night in his sleep, Noel scratched a mosquito bite, and we woke in the morning to see that his foot was bleeding. I enjoyed the reversal of roles as I nursed his wound, disinfecting and bandaging the abrasion. But the strap of his sandal cut into the sore, and with another walk in the countryside it became infected. After sitting with an elevated foot for three days, he made a suggestion: *Let's drive to Florence tomorrow, okay?*

We decided to roller-coaster our way on back roads that would take us through small villages and keep us close to the poppies and sunflowers. Since my chemotherapy injections, I had made a point of drinking ten glasses of water a day to cleanse my kidneys and liver, and to ensure that I would never again experience the swollen, fuzzy, suffocating tongue that accompanies serious dehydration. This task had been made simple by the Tuscan heat and the availability of mineral water. But the consequence was always the same. I told Noel I would soon have to make a pee stop.

After ten minutes of sitting very still, I contemplated the expression *gird your loins*. A stirring in the folds of my white skirt caught my eye. Crawling up my skirt was a large black spider with a hairy tail. *Scorpion!* I yelled. *Stop! Oh my god! Do something, do something!* My voice was an octave higher and several decibels louder than usual. *Sweetie, there's nowhere to pull off,* Noel coaxed. Later we would both take credit for knocking the scorpion off my skirt and onto the floor. I loosened my safety belt and arched back over the seat with some vague plan of jumping out while the car sped along. As I pulled at the handle, I felt the scorpion on the back of my bare thigh and froze.

Suddenly the car had stopped and I had tumbled out. My feet hit the roadside, dislodging the scorpion, which began to saunter off, indignant at being uprooted. Noel's large brown sandal came down on the intruder. *Are you all right?* he asked, stroking my hair. *How come you killed it?* I sniveled. We leaned against the Lancia and laughed until we gasped for breath.

On our next outing, we learned that the gods have other ways of extracting their dues from tourists. On our way south to Perugia, the road offered a special challenge to drivers who need glasses. Our car disappeared into dark tunnels that run through outcroppings of rock. The heavenly architect of these hills and the earthly one who created the tunnels each had a sense of humor. No sooner had our eyes adjusted than we burst into the white Tuscan sun, blind as the bats we saw each night at dusk.

Noel had recently turned fifty. Although he has perfect reading vision, he confessed (*after* I agreed to marry him) to a need for distance-vision glasses. While he sped along, eyes on the road, I was given two tasks. The first was to decipher road signs with my perfect distance vision. The second, which required my reading glasses, was to match the names on the signs to the names on the map. Noel, meantime, to see in the dark, had to whip off the sun visors attached to his glasses. As he pulled at the visor, he had to ensure that his featherweight glasses stayed attached to his ears. Between us we kept up a constant arm motion, like marching puppets gone mad, elbows bashing, vocabulary disintegrating as we raised and lowered our glasses to look through eyes that had left their youth to memory.

Perhaps this was why we had felt so drawn to each other in the first place. Together we had perfect sight. The problem was we had never before had to use *both* sets of eyes for *both* distances. I wondered if I had gone into remission only to be mutilated by an oncoming tunnel as my eyes adjusted, travelling at speeds that gave no respect to age. Patting the floor in search of my reading glasses, fearing the return of the scorpion, I heard Noel brag, *I can steer with my knees* as he removed the visor with both hands. We arrived in Perugia with the realization that we may have married without knowing each other well enough.

Whenever we felt stressed, we bought another map. After being jocular with a storekeeper who told us we had parked in the *carabiniere* stall, I was left behind to pay for the map while Noel ventured into the chaos of Perugia to find a legitimate spot. As the city swallowed up the Lancia, my stomach told me I would never see him again. I tried to be philosophical and reminded myself that I had lived many years and traveled many cities before meeting him. I bought the *Herald Tribune* and ordered *caffè latte* and a breakfast pastry. But after I had read the newspaper and watched people go by, my eyes began to search for the long tall body and shiny pate I thought of as home. As I peered over pedestrians, hawkers, scooters, motorcycles, cars, and buses, the noise and heat began to close in. I tried to consider the beauties of times past, the small considerations Noel had brought to my life, our moments of grace.

I locked myself in a dim *toletta* and promised my reflection in the mirror that I would use every skill I had to find my beloved. I envisioned wandering the streets of Perugia for days, looking for a lime-green Lancia. After I had cooled my body to a mild fever, I opened the door. Noel was right there, grinning like a happy hound. *How did you find me?* I asked. *Oh,* he said, *I have my ways.*

A week later, as we waited to catch the train, I noticed the electronic board was blank. I read my half of the *Herald Tribune* as people rushed about shouting at one another or stood dazed by the tracks. The noise seemed frenzied, but I reasoned it was the beginning of siesta and everyone was headed home. The repeated word *sciopero* meant nothing to me. Suddenly Noel tossed his half of the paper aside and sprang to his feet. I tried to keep up as he raced to the information desk. I found him talking with agitation to the clerk. Then he was off again, shouting for me to follow. I was responsible for only one small bottle of water, a fanny pack, and my half of the newspaper, whereas he carried the knapsack of books and clothes, but the length of my legs is no match for his and he soon outpaced me. I wondered why everyone was so frantic, jogging through the record-breaking heat.

Elizabeth! Over here! Hurry!

I could hear Noel, but not find his face. Usually this was not a problem as he stood taller than most Italians. I finally discovered him dangling out the door of a train on a distant track. He reached down to grab me as the train began to shuttle forward. *It's a rail strike*, he yelled. *Move it!* Cancer allowed me to obey without shame; illness may teach patients the impotence of wealth and power and beauty, but it puts a premium on trust. I leapt into his arms with all the abandon of a middle-aged bride.

On our final morning, when we said good-bye to Sharon and Dan, I felt as though we had been in Tuscany forever and yet as though the holiday had been a brief dream. On the bridge, we paused to look back. It occurred to me that I might never have the privilege of returning. I narrowed into finite time for a moment, and then expanded into the eternity of sunflowers and poppies that stretched from Tuscany to Rome.

At our hotel in Rome, a rattling cage took us up the five floors to our room. A rotating Metro strike kept us there for half a day. I had begun to suffer from back pain and numb legs, and I feared the many things that pain and numbness can portend. When I fell asleep, pain woke me; my numb legs would not carry me to the bathroom. My heart stuttered with a desire to be home. I tried to concentrate on all the innocent backaches I had known over the years, after a vigorous squash game or a frenzied attempt to finish painting an entire room in one evening. I was terrified, and for the first time in our relationship, I could not be alone with my terror.

When I woke Noel, he thought carefully. He asked what I was carrying in the fanny pack I had strapped to my waist. He went to where I had stashed it and groaned when he pulled out my camera. *What the hell is this doing in there?* He began to toss the contents on the bed. *You knew it was there,* I argued. *And this?* he said, *And this?* repeating the question with each revelation. I had worn the pack back-to-front to avoid pickpockets, and so I would not have to take it off when I sat down. My lower back muscles had done all the lugging. *What's this?* he repeated, dragging out my flashlight and notebook. I shrugged. When I failed again to make my legs move forward, he offered to carry my stuff in his knapsack. *It's not the same,* I complained. *Damn right!* he agreed. I fell asleep listening to Noel enumerate what I was allowed to carry: my tissue, a comb, sunglasses....

When I woke in late afternoon, my knees propped up by extra blankets, my backache was gone. We roused ourselves to catch the now-running Metro and then strolled lovely streets toward the Trevi Fountain. Long gone are the days when a few passersby loiter about pristine waters. To my highly sensitive nose, the *purest water in Italy* smelled of chlorine, and people circled the area in rows as though in a stadium watching a drama. Noel tossed a coin over his shoulder, and I wondered if his wish had involved my health or an Italian sports car. As I turned to watch my own coin fall, I remembered years ago wishing to return to Rome. Now, I could not imagine wanting more than what I had.

As we were returning to our hotel, we ran headlong into a wedding party led along the streets by the bride and groom. She wore a long, elaborate white dress with the traditional veil to express her virtue. He wore a cream-colored military suit with a sheathed sword hanging from his belt as a sign of manliness. Guests filled the streets for as far as we could see, following the couple from cathedral to reception. When the bride stopped to adjust her dress, I captured the moment on film. As the camera rewound itself, I realized why I had saved my wish at the fountain. I caught the eye of the bride, and I wished for her a holiday in the green spaciousness of Canada.

The gods seem intent on reminding people of their good fortune by giving them contrast. On the plane home, I slipped off my oxygen mask at dinner time, just as the woman behind us returned from the bathroom, awash with the pungent odor of perfume. With each breath I began to feel more nauseated until finally I crawled back into my mask. During the long landing I had to close off the tank, and I became nauseated enough for the attendant to offer me a wheelchair. I declined, knowing I would feel infinitely better away from the offending smell. We bend our senses to the rose because we trust that it keeps its perfume subtle.

Home. The Gulf Islands float evergreen on a blue background as we look down from the plane. Their familiarity makes me feel substantial in a self-satisfying way. Among my own deck flowers, I startle a hummingbird and breathe the early-morning air. In bare feet, I wander around the disarray of the garden, listening to a woodpecker tapping in someone else's tree. In spite of my cancer, I feel privileged. I consider once again how much I want to live a long life and to be buried in the earth or sprinkled over the water in this place I call home. Two gray squirrels chase each other to the middle of the lawn where they collide and chatter into each other's fur before they catch sight of me and bound up our apple tree. Making a U-turn midway, they scurry back down, stopping and starting on their way toward the blackberry bushes. Their days have just begun and hope comes naturally to them.

Inside the house, sun pours summer through the windows. I see that robins have nested for the first time outside our front window. The birds have chosen the inner sanctum of an evergreen whose branches touch our exterior walls. Their hiding place can be seen only from our living room, which was uninhabited when they chose the spot. The dark bowl of mud and twigs sits in a space that captures a shaft of both morning and evening sun. I stand very still, looking down on their nest. As the female rises from her brooding position, I glimpse three blue ovals in the basket. At the same moment that she exposes her eggs, the red-breasted male returns with a worm clutched in his beak like a writhing piece of spaghetti.

Within a day, two chicks appear, beak first. The next day, the third hatches. Their beaks remain perfectly still and open for long periods, as though they were posing for an artist. They continue through the day to yawn for sustenance. Each morning they have grown noticeably until one day their necks reach over the top of the nest. Sibling rivalry erupts each time a parent returns with food. On the off chance that I might disturb them, I discipline myself to look no more than three times a day, but it is a little like resisting *gelati* – sometimes I cheat. As I watch the parents nervously ensuring the survival of their young, I remember the birds of Tuscany and think of how all birds are the same and yet each is unique. I sense that the robins share this precious knowing with me. In my own corner of the universe, I have uncovered a sacred moment.

Home. I cannot avoid the terrifying thought that my return

coincides with my third six-month checkup at the clinic. On appointment day I awaken before the robins with a quickening of my heart. It seems hours before Noel stirs, opens his eyes, and smiles. Yet before I can still my fear, the automatic doors of the clinic open to pass my flesh and bones into the hands of the oncologist. He is a summer replacement for my female chemotherapist, Heidi; I feel agitated by the change but quickly grow to respect him. He is a direct and thorough man who satisfies my curiosity with informative comments as he examines my spine, breasts, and stomach. He tells me I appear to be in good health before sending me off to the adjoining building with a requisition for a chest x-ray and a blood test. On my way to the laboratory, I suddenly find myself instead in my car driving home. As promised, I phone Noel. I tell him all appears well, and I hear joy in his assurances: *We'll die in our nineties with our boots on.*

Each time I think of the laboratory requisition in my handbag, I return to the window and watch the baby robins. I think of all my foolish debaucheries in Italy and fear overtakes me. Perhaps I deserve to die for the disrespect I have shown my body. At dusk I see the mother robin plump down like a tea cozy over her offspring. I remember my own mother's vigilance, juggling with courage and dignity three children and cancer.

On the sixth day after my visit, I finally go to the laboratory. Back home after the tests, I phone the clinic to confess my delay, then wait for the doctor's call. He phones the next afternoon to say everything looks fine, *the test results are good.* There is *bad news and good news*, he tells me, as though sharing a joke. The bad news is that more young women are being diagnosed each year with lung cancer – by young, he means women in their forties and fifties. The good news, he says, is *they're still coming back after five and six years.*

Soon the baby robins are as big as their parents, distinguishable only by their speckled breasts. Two overflow the nest and the third sits motionless on a branch above them. A day later, the nest is empty; even the mother does not return. I feel bereft until the kettle whistles for my attention. Through the kitchen window, in the back yard I glimpse the beating of wings and a spray of water that arcs from the birdbath onto the deck. The baby robins are learning to bathe. In the enchantment of a summer morning, I gather my future in the joy of their ablutions.

✤ 10 ✤

Bounding
Toward Wisdom

I began writing this book with my old Airedale, Chance, snooz-
ing close by. In her sixteenth year, she forced me to get up and
out each day of my cancer treatments regardless of how I felt.
We did a slow dance toward the water for the sake of her aging
bladder and my battered body. Gingerly placing one foot in front
of the other, we reached a place where, with her stiff joints and my
feeble flesh, we could scamper about in a modest replica of our
former vigor.

Having exceeded the normal life span of an Airedale, Chance
made me wonder whether she would understand what had
become of her companion if I happened upon death before she
did. For me she had embodied the dual magic of hope and loyalty,
sticking by me through the deaths of family and friends, keeping
close as I stumbled through my second divorce, standing guard by
the front door as I slept, or sitting patiently outside a store until I
returned, always expecting the wait would be worth the reunion.
As a final bonus she adapted like a puppy to the affections of my
new husband. When she died, I imagined I would never own
another dog. As a cancer patient I felt that a puppy should not be
left to mourn the loss of its mistress. But why, I pondered, should
cancer be the only reality to which I gave credence?

Chance had been my third puppy. I had picked my first from a litter of three in my neighbor's kitchen when I was nine years old. I was supposed to watch the births, but I was in school when the puppies came to rest on an old blanket by a heat duct. No matter, I named mine Boots and, after six weeks, I carried home her squirming black body with its white paws. My mother told me we would breed her and watch the birth of our own puppies. But one morning a year later we got up to find three whimpering ovals of wet fur snuggled against her tummy and tugging milk from her swollen nipples.

She had tricked my mother once before, on our two-week summer holiday in Banff. Our green 1951 Chevrolet was already packed with three children, one grandmother, two parents, and a trunk full of camping gear. Having sneaked onto the floor of the back seat, Boots kept a low profile, so low that my parents agreed to take her on our trailer holiday to the Okanagan the following year. There she bit a boy who kicked her, and the warden said she had to be put down. My father disappeared with the uniformed official and returned later with the dog. When we clustered around to ask how he had saved Boots, he just put his index finger to his puckered lips: *Shshsh.*

Boots was killed by a man who did not see her zip under his front wheel when she attempted to follow my younger sister to school. In 1957, on Elphinstone Street in Regina, the driver had to meet the eyes of an entire family as we blocked noon-hour traffic in an effort to protect our seven-year-old dog from further humiliation. Finally my father picked her up from a pool of blood and told us she wouldn't have felt a thing. He laid her on the grass in such a way that we could not see the crushed side of her skull. The following Saturday, he made a small wooden cross to take into the countryside where we buried her in a wheat field.

I remember my astonishment at my father's tears. *A dog needs to know who the boss is,* he used to tell me. Mother would have her say too. She would give the dog away, she said, if I kept forgetting to brush her and wash her bowl. *There's more to a dog than playing with it,* she had told me. But she cried for days when Boots died. The rest of the family moved about in stunned silence. *Your mother is not usually like this,* my father explained, his hand on her shoulder. Mother sniveled into her lace-edged handkerchief, *She sat at my feet after my operation.* Once Mother came to her senses, she revealed my younger sister's part in the death. *Your sister feels really badly,* she whispered to me. Until then it had not occurred to me to blame my sister. We never got another dog. As far as I was concerned, it would have been disloyal.

My first husband knew how I felt about owning a dog. He and I had met when I was fifteen and he was seventeen. Emboldened by marriage and university, he came home one day with a persuasive tale. Walking back from the store he had discovered a collie puppy that would be put to sleep if we didn't rescue it. I reacted with astonishment. *What are we going to do with a dog in Europe?* I asked, reminding him of our extended trip just fourteen months away. He bargained for a hearing. *Just come and see her; maybe we can think up something.* But I was adamant: *Who's going to look after her?*

There on the front steps behind a broken fence sat a twelve-year-old boy crying as though his baseball glove had been chewed by a lawn mower. A three-month-old collie sat beside him, craning her fragile nose up to lick his dripping cheeks. *What's the matter?* I asked. The boy explained between sobs that his father had returned with the drunken resolve that *no dog's going to piss inside his goddamn house.* He told us his father was going to kill the puppy when he woke up. *I got her with my newspaper money,* he gulped, as though payment in full should solve the problems of alcoholism and an untrained bladder. *How much?* I asked. *Five dollars,* he said. The puppy watched us from the dark pools of her eyes, emphasized by nature's outline of charcoal against her blond coat. *We'll take her to live in our yard,* I said, *and my husband will give you five dollars to show your dad.* The look in the boy's eyes was worth the price of our two Friday movie tickets. In a loving tone, my husband agreed: *You can own her, but she'll live at our place.* With the trust of young things, neither the boy nor the dog objected when my husband swept up the puppy and carried her off.

We arrived home to discover a friend on our doorstep, a physicist who had arrived from England to work at the university. He always sipped his beer with the same salutation – *Here's to Fred!* – and the habit had spread to our kitchen. So it came to be that we named Fred. While she grew into a collie-cross version of Lassie, her first master and his family were evicted from their rented house. We never saw the boy again; the following spring we went to Europe. The physicist moved into our house with his new bride, and they bought Fred a kitten to play with while they were at work.

Six months later, when we arrived back in Canada, the physicist and his wife were adamant about their right to own the dog. We felt guilty and confused listening to them sob as they picked up their cat and said good-bye. Fred turned her face to the wall and refused to look at me. It wasn't until hours later that she came padding through the dark to sniff my arm from fingertips to shoulder and back down again. Finally her tail began to wag slowly and she snuggled down on the rug beside me. I stroked her head and she let out an anguished howl before she curled up to sleep. From then on we took her everywhere, even to Cambridge. Pregnant, propped between the emergency brake and the crowded back seat of our MG, she lay silent for three long days as we drove from Manitoba to Massachusetts.

At the age of twenty-seven, I was finally able to see how live things come into the world. Seven live things entered our two-room apartment in Cambridge in the hours before dawn. Fred gave birth to the first puppy on our buffalo rug at the end of our bed. I picked up this warm and slippery life, and Fred followed us to the kennel my husband had built on the far side of the room. The puppy was not destined to be lonely. Its siblings kept arriving for four hours. We watched Fred's agitation over the birth that turned out to be her last. My husband wanted to save her discomfort by helping, but when I saw him take scissors from the drawer, I persuaded him she knew what she was doing. She stood up and shook her hind end until the puppy dropped out, wrapped in a glistening sack. Fred nipped the sack open and licked the puppy's stomach. Eventually it breathed on its own and stumbled over to mingle with the other wet flesh wriggling beside the mother. Only then did Fred struggle to her feet, climb over the puppies' barricade, and trot down two flights of stairs to go outside. When she returned, she counted her litter with her nose.

For the next six weeks our two rooms were filled with the sound of our laughter. My husband decided to keep all seven puppies. *We can't have eight dogs!* I argued. *Why not? Architects earn lots of money,* he said, as though expense would be the only change in having eight large dogs to squeeze into an MG. Although I could not come up with a logic he found satisfactory, I advertised them. Soon only three puppies remained – the tri-colored one my husband called Cleopatra and was determined to adopt, a blond puppy we had named Goldie, and of course Blackie, the puppy we loved the way people love helpless things. This last birth had produced a physically strong but slow-witted puppy who watched and waited with his tail wagging in apparent delight at all he saw.

A Harvard student from India came to take Goldie away. His landlady had been in mourning since her dog collided with a car. I was hesitant. My neighbor, an anthropologist, was doing a doctorate on the eating customs of families in India and he had told me Indians did not include dogs in their family life. *Never?* I asked. *It's just not part of their culture*, he said. But the student's eyes were kind and Goldie licked his ear when he held her. Cleo was inconsolable when they left. She refused to move for the rest of the day, and then as suddenly as she had given up on life, she rebounded to tackle Blackie in an effort to teach him how to play with more zest.

Someone interrupted their antics by knocking on the apartment door. Two rather shy parents came in with an adult daughter whose face told me she suffered from Down syndrome: *Would you consider giving our daughter one of your puppies?* the father asked. When I passed Blackie to the eager girl, she was speechless. She looked first to her mother and then to her father as they reassured her. She forgot to look back and wave as she had promised, but I felt content that she and Blackie would work out a companionship that the parents would safeguard from those less sensitive.

When my husband and I returned to Canada, we had two big collies crowded into the MG, one shedding her golden hair and the other her tri-colored coat. When the sorrow of our inability to conceive eventually destroyed our marriage, Cleo went to live with my husband's parents. Fred and I were initially separated when my husband moved to Calgary and I moved to Vancouver, but when he visited me two years later, I coaxed him to let me have her again. She watched him drive off in his Alfa Romeo before bolting out the door, her back legs pumping in the increasing distance as I called to her. When I found her exhausted at the curb and carried her back to my apartment, she put her head in the corner, having for one brief day assumed that my husband and I were reunited.

After two years apart, Fred and I were inseparable, going off to graduate school at U.B.C. and discovering British Columbia together. No landlord ever argued against her. In fact, one landlady, a doctor, had married and become pregnant just before her fortieth birthday. When she miscarried, she made a slow recovery from despair and would speak to no one except the collie, who seemed to listen to her with all the compassion of one who had lost part of her family too. The next year my landlady again became pregnant. This time she lasted into her fourth month before losing her baby. Afterward, she would wander like a sleepwalker into the garden and spend long hours talking to Fred about things that the dog kept confidential. At the end of her reclusion, she used her professional clout to take over a hospital bed for several months and produce a perfect baby girl and then another. As the mother grew younger and her children grew older, Fred contented herself to watch from the distance of our doorstep. She had just given me my first lesson in the healing power of flesh that barks.

My second husband learned to love the collie because, unlike me, she was always glad to see him. She did not mind whether he arrived home on the same day he left or whether he was sober. In fact, she adapted to his happy-go-lucky ways and left with him for a few hours one night when, as a woman scorned, I lost my temper and accidentally locked her outside with him. Fred also gained his respect when we took her in our camper for a two-day mountain climb. In the parking lot, we saw a sign that read *No dogs on the trails.* Given the squirrels and bears along the climb, the request was reasonable. *We'll have to tie her up outside the camper,* my husband suggested. *I don't want to leave her helpless against wild animals,* I argued. Home was a long drive away, so we stood there looking for a solution. *How about if I promise to install a new rug in the camper as soon as we get back?* I held my breath. *It's your call,* my husband laughed. We left her with water and food before we locked the camper door. When we came down the mountain two days later and opened the door, the dog shot out *over* the shoulder of my six-foot two-inch husband and into the bush without greeting us. The food bowls were empty and the rug was spotless.

Without a whimper, Fred died in a bed of flowers as darkness spread over the Okanagan one August evening in her fourteenth year. My intuition had peaked to an inner scream for no discernible cause, and I had gone to search for her with a flashlight. For the last half of her life, she had remained a link between me and my first husband, a connection that covered the miles and the years. *She must be unconscious,* I told my second husband when he found me on my knees. *She's dead, luv,* he said, pointing out her stiffening limbs. *She's cold,* I whimpered into the warm evening. He carried her in to spend the night on the living-room rug where I could look at her and absorb the loss.

Fred's heart had mended after the loss of her brief youthful master, and again after her separation from my first husband, but by morning it was clear her heart would not mend again. *Will you dig her a grave right there?* I asked my husband. I pointed to a place near our prolific apricot tree. *Get real,* he protested – *that's rock!* Our house sat on a mountainside, surrounded by forest. There was nowhere else I could plant Fred to protect her from the wild animals who would dig her up. *I'll never ask another thing of you,* I lied. He waited for the hardware store to open and returned with a pickax that he swung repeatedly until he had dug a space big enough to hold a collie. *What about her basket?* I asked. *I may be crazy, but I'm not stupid,* he said, putting down the ax and picking up a beer. But he reconsidered and returned to dig for the rest of the morning. We wept together as we covered her with earth and stone. The kindness he showed me that day lives on.

In the spring that followed Fred's death, my mother and my second husband arranged that he would drive to Vancouver and choose a puppy from a litter of Airedales she had found in the newspaper. I listened reluctantly to him list the advantages of an Airedale – good watchdogs, fabulous with children, no hair to vacuum. We lived in a remote cabin on a mountainside where a watchdog was a valuable commodity. We had reason to believe we would have at least one child before my fortieth birthday. And anyone who has owned a collie deserves a break from finding long blond dog hairs in the salad.

The breeders were a retired couple who ran a theater in Vancouver. In their kitchen, a gyrating mass of warm bodies rushed toward the cupboard as the woman rustled a paper bag of dry chow to distract them. One puppy broke free and bounded over to lick the toes that protruded from my summer sandals before she tried to leap up my leg to be held. *I want this one,* I laughed, picking her up to see her pink belly and large black nose. *She thinks I taste better than lunch.* The woman looked up from the eleven churning puppies. *I'm sorry,* she said. *Every one of them has been paid for and labeled with its owner's name.* I checked its name tag: *"For Elizabeth."*

When the puppy vomited in the car on the way home, I still thought she was adorable. I told my husband the mess would clean up easily with a bit of sudsy water. *Puppy vomit doesn't stink,* I said. When a small boy asked to hold her while we ate our picnic lunch, I said, *Not right now, she's too frightened,* as she squirmed to get out of my arms and into his. When she cried from the bathroom on her first night away from her siblings, I opened the door and let her lie on the rug by my side of the bed. She slept soundly as long as my hand dangled over the side. *I guess you like her,* my husband said.

In spite of the reputation of Airedales as watchdogs, Chance adored everyone. I named her during what I thought was an inspired moment. In one of Susanna Moodie's pioneer journals, she tells of a visiting woodsman with a big dog named Chance, and of how this hunter had mourned the loss of his companion when it was shot for killing eight sheep. Moodie recalled her visitor saying that he *would have restored the sheep fourfold* if he had been allowed to keep his beloved dog. I resolved that a well-trained dog was a long-lived dog. But in Chance's ninth year, my theory was put to the test when she bit a boy who came between her and a Doberman.

By this time we lived in Victoria, and my second marriage was in disarray. In a house full of tension, the Airedale paced from room to room trying to distract us. To work off my hurt and my husband's anger, we dug out our tennis rackets and crossed to the park. He insisted I tie up the dog; I argued that she never strayed, but a sign supported his opinion: *All dogs on leash.* While we batted the ball at each other, a twelve-year-old boy lay down on the grass and stretched over to hug the dog who was straining toward him at the end of her leash. A Doberman lunged at them, and the boy came out of the fray with blood pouring from his cheek. The people with the Doberman disappeared, and we rushed the boy home.

He was a lonely child whose father had left and whose mother was in California temporarily. The stepfather was reluctant to call an ambulance or to go with it when we called one. I phoned the hospital to ask that the boy be given at my expense whatever plastic surgery was necessary. I took a deep breath, then, and called the pound to turn Chance in for biting a child. When the official arrived, he looked at Chance resting in the summer sun and gave me some advice. *Get her a license.* I never saw him again, but that evening I visited the boy and assured him that Chance would live and that his tidy scar would give him a great story to tell his friends.

This was not the first lesson Chance had taught me about survival. When I had taken her to have her first puppy shots, the vet had diagnosed her as having a diseased liver. He said that a damaged liver was the cause of her small size and that I would save her considerable discomfort if I put her to sleep. For a price, he would do it for me. Instead I spent my money on long-distance phone bills, calling all the other owners of puppies in her litter of eight females and four males. The answers I got were all the same: the female puppies weighed in at forty-four pounds, the males slightly more. They were bred to be fragile.

When Chance reached her first heat, my first husband, with whom I remained friends, bought a male Airedale in Calgary to mate with the female Airedale that my second husband had bought for me in Vancouver. In spite of Cougar's registration papers, his brawn, and his beauty, Chance refused him. She simply sat down and barked instead. Both men pondered the notion that I had taught her by example. After having Chance spayed, our female vet told me that the dog's ovaries and womb had been unusually small and strangely entwined with other organs.

After the loss of her womb, Chance showed no signs of discomfort and was soon well enough to play with the neighbor's German shepherd puppy, Sasha. They roamed the hills to scout for porcupine, always losing their battles with the wild. I rescued Chance with her big black nose and her leg joints full of quills. She could do no more than cry from the mountain top. As I carried her down, I slipped on some loose shale, and we both rolled to the bottom. She was back in the forest the next day while I sat in the tub massaging my bruises.

Just before Chance's third birthday, my husband was offered a promotion that required our moving to Victoria. I refused to go at first, having found myself a permanent position and fearing that our irreconcilable differences would simply travel with us. No one, it seemed, considered it a deprivation for a woman to leave her hard-won faculty post to follow her husband, although many thought I was being difficult when I refused to move again in the years to come. As my husband drove off alone and I promised to follow in three months, Chance bounded out of the forest and licked the tears that dripped from my face.

When my husband came back with a moving truck at Christmas, Sasha, the neighbor's dog, sat beside the truck as we filled it with furniture and locked the doors. Snow had almost obliterated her, and I looked back as we pulled out of the driveway. *Do you think we could take her too?* I asked. *Do you want the police down our necks?* he answered. I pondered arguing that he risked the wrath of the police when he drank and drove, but I knew my suggestion would not win Sasha's escape.

Chance's days changed from racing around an acreage outside

Kelowna to sitting behind a chain-link fence in Victoria. My days changed from meetings with college students and colleagues to the empty hours of a jobless woman. Chance, however, made friends with the old man next door who had suffered repeated heart attacks and was glad for some company. In the fall I was offered a temporary job at a local college, and the next year I was offered a sessional position at the University of Victoria. My second husband and I found a house within blocks of the water where Chance could run along the tide line and chase sticks in the cold water. After she leapt the hedge to introduce herself to our new neighbor, I went over to apologize.

Propped up by crutches, the neighbor, Noel's cousin, welcomed me. She was a dwarf I called Little Lynn (to distinguish her from my younger sister). She asked if she could keep the dog while my husband and I were at work. I hesitated in a moment of possessiveness, then looked at the baking on her kitchen counter and the gentle friends around the table of her cooperative house. From then on, to the horror of her crabby cat, I left Chance on the neighbor's doorstep in the morning and whistled for her when I arrived home. The S.P.C.A. agreed that she was free to roam from one yard to another as long as we had both addresses on her collar. Surrounded by young nurses who took her walking, Chance lived in uninterrupted glory until she was eleven years old.

One November night just after my second husband left us, Chance woke me with her frenzied gouging at the front door. I had trained her to be discreet – no sidewalks, no rugs, no neighborhood yards, and no door scratching. She also had to be quiet until I was up. Because she had obeyed, I thought her frenzy meant she was about to upchuck her dinner. But when I opened the door, she leapt over the bushes and onto the next porch where she began defacing the neighbor's door. I grabbed my housecoat with one hand and her collar with the other and dragged her home. As I crawled back into bed the clock said 2:10. Before I had the covers pulled up, she was back at the front door, working to carve a hole through the heavy wood. Such desperation in a dog considered elderly by Airedale standards caused me to open the door once again. Once again she leaped off the stairway and onto the neighbor's porch. I dragged her home a second time.

In the morning, Chance was reluctant to leave the house for our exercise. An ambulance sat outside. It had come to fetch Chance's other mistress, her handicapped friend of seven years. Little Lynn had suffered a massive heart attack at the age of forty-eight, still in her wheelchair. She had died quietly, not even reaching for her call-bell. The ambulance drivers estimated she had died around 2 A.M. One of the nurses asked if I had seen Little Lynn's cat. He and Chance had stalked each other for years, hissing and growling. I wondered if Chance, in her sorrow, had crushed him with those mighty bear-bating jaws. Then I realized that the dog was missing as well. When a nurse found them, they were curled up on the same pillow in a darkened closet. When we tried to separate them, they refused to be parted.

The cat went to live out her life with five dogs on a farm. Chance went daily to sit on Lynn's front porch as though making some statement about loyalty. When new people moved in, I asked them to give the dog a few sharp commands, assuring them she would respond to their scolding and would not need punishing further. *Could she stay with us?* they asked. *Just while you're at work,* the young wife coaxed. *I'm here studying most of the day.* I hesitated. What if they fed her candy while she befriended their Siamese cat? But the two pets moved freely between our houses, and by the time the couple moved, the dog was too old to mind solitude.

Old or not, Chance still had a few tricks left to teach me. Each year I took her to a veterinarian for her shots. The vet told me that she had grown a lump on her side. *Feel that*, he suggested as he poked under her ribs. *I can't feel anything unusual*, I said. *It's her spleen*, he told me. *She needs it out as soon as possible – enlarged and possibly killing her.* I knew something about spleens. My mother had lost hers after the chemotherapy treatments that ravaged her organs but bought her time. She had won twelve palliative years by parting with one kidney and her spleen. She comforted me by saying a body could function in apparent good health without a spleen: *Football players do it all the time.*

There's no swelling there, I argued, picking the dog off the table and walking through the crowded office with an enormous animal, struggling to keep us both from falling while I sobbed into her coat. *My dad just died,* I shouted back at the vet, overwhelmed by a female logic few men can grasp. A woman in the waiting room opened the door for me. *You're beautiful*, she said. *You and your dog.* When I got home I phoned a traveling veterinarian. He could find nothing wrong except for the rapid panting that could indicate a heart problem.

When I arrived home from work in Chance's thirteenth year and she could not even get up to greet me, I decided to let her die with dignity. I carried her outside, laid her on the grass, and stroked her head while I talked about how much joy she had brought me. She struggled to her feet in response, inspiring me to hustle her to the animal hospital. My new vet diagnosed a virus and stayed up through the night to give the dog a blood transfusion. I returned to the dark house, wondering how Chance would endure the hospital without me. When I fetched her two days later, she had befriended half the staff and barely noticed my arrival. When this vet moved to England, she recommended another who looked after Chance into her old age, medicating away the dog's incontinence and giving me free phone visits to instruct me on how to keep food in an aging dog's stomach when my cancer surgery and treatments had left me unable to drive.

Noel expressed no great love for dogs when we began our relationship. I convinced him that Chance would sleep on his indoor porch on my weekends in Vancouver, and he would simply have to accept her on the weekends he was to visit me. He saw this as fair, and the dog seemed to understand the rules of alternating privileges. As the months passed and their friendship grew, I suggested that he was spoiling her. *Dogs need a little consistency*, I reminded him, jealous that Chance had thumped her tail on my arrival home from shopping but had stayed snugged up beside *my* new man. *She's consistently spoiled,* he said before they turned their attention back to each other. Feeling ignored, I graded papers until Noel came out to say he would pick up groceries for dinner. After the door closed, I called the dog. When she didn't respond, I looked out the front window. Her chin was propped on the leather curve of the backrest of Noel's convertible.

By the time cancer had come to live with us, Noel had moved to Victoria and we three formed a trio bent on keeping me alive. He and Chance kept me company through my diagnosis, surgery, chemotherapy, radiation, and recovery. The most astonishing thing Chance gave me during my illness was not the impetus to get out of bed when I was in pain or nauseated. It was the knowledge that our friends, even those who seemed indifferent to dogs, were willing to walk her whenever I was indisposed and Noel was away. The woman who took the most pains to see that Chance was fed, watered, and walked was Trudy, who became my bridesmaid when Noel and I married. Despite four children, a full-time job, and a singing career, she carried the dog up and down stairs that four arthritic legs could no longer maneuver with ease.

From November 1994, when I was diagnosed with pneumonia, to November 1995, when I went from a serious illness to a serious attempt to survive, Chance and I kept a constant vigil over one another. It was a year after my treatments had ended that Noel caught me carrying her up and down the stairs. Until autumn I had kept this effort a secret – a lie by omission. Noel had assumed that if he got up a half hour early to walk Chance and then repeated their walk after work, she could make it down the stairs unaided for her and my daily walk together. But her bladder was beyond the help of medication when she slept. I knew what the consequence would be if such a large dog were unable to get outside. *She's lived a long life*, Noel told me. *It's your turn to be babied now.* I ignored him and carried her down the steps and into the car to visit the vet. *She's confused,* the vet told me. Confused or not, I thought, she's still Chance to me. Old, blind, deaf, and arthritic, she tangled herself in some tree branches the next day and couldn't back up the few inches necessary to free herself. I watched her stand immobile as the unspeakable truth closed in.

I went to bed without speaking to Noel, although I had been the one to make the appointment at the animal hospital. At 2:30 A.M. I awoke alone. *What are you doing up?* I asked when I found him in the living room. *I didn't want her to spend her last night alone,* he explained. Of all the sweet nothings I have heard over the years, these words touched home. I snuggled up to him on the couch: *Why don't you go back to bed and I'll stay up for the second shift?* I spent the long night searching through Chance's puppy pictures from the Okanagan to her days with Little Lynn, making a photo collage. By morning I was laughing at memories of her escapades: Getting her head stuck in a plant pot. Leaping wet with saltwater into a police car when the officers got out to stretch their legs. Bounding *through* the new screen door to learn that my second husband's charm hid a powerful temper. Watching him build a fence and then leaping over it. She slept trustingly by my chair as I meandered through our years together.

In the morning I let her do something she had never been allowed to do before. She sat on my knee in the car, wrapped in a blanket even though an Airedale is hardy enough to withstand most winter storms, even though I had for years argued that dogs should be afforded the dignity of being dogs and not pseudo persons, and even though she was too big to fit easily between the emergency brake and the door. Perhaps she knew something was up because she nuzzled into my collar as we drove to the hospital.

When the vet's needle slipped beneath her skin, and recognition faded into a cataract haze, I thanked her for her friendship and promised I would sprinkle her ashes along the path we had walked. I last saw her stretched out on her blanket. Noel and I left with our chins up before we sat in the car and sobbed, unable to stem our tears for longer than either of us later cared to admit. Chance's ashes sat for a year in a pottery jar on the fridge, reminding me that I had to walk for both of us and prove that *not* carrying her up and down the stairs was indeed good for my health.

The day before we were to sprinkle Chance's ashes, just before the anniversary of her death, someone knocked on our door. A woman stood there with a tall cinnamon-colored poodle with brown silken ears. She introduced herself as Cindy and her dog as Forget-Me-Not. She told me she had met Noel one night as he had carried our Airedale across the road. *I knew he was a dog lover,* she exclaimed. I resisted telling her of the forty-five years he had ignored the canine population or thought of it as something that fools endured. She wanted to share with us the name of the woman who bred these blond poodles on her beautiful farm in the Annapolis Valley. I vaguely remembered Noel telling me this story, but cancer treatments and losing Chance had fogged my memory. I did remember telling him that I didn't want a silly poodle with pompoms as an excuse for a dog. He had assured me that the dog was good looking and obedient, with no pompoms anywhere. Forget-Me-Not stood silently by while Cindy and I talked. With the timing of an acrobat, she told me she had been called by the breeder in Nova Scotia to say that a new litter of poodle puppies had been born and were named after cities. One was named Victoria.

Noel was reading when I interrupted. *Guess what I bought to help us keep me in remission!* His face took a serious turn. *Not a dog, I hope.* He kept his eyes on mine. *Remember your cardinal rule when we decided to live together? No decisions without consultations,* he reminded me. *I didn't buy her,* I assured him. *I just ordered her.* That's when he got picky. *Her?* Before things grew too difficult, I made a suggestion: *We could always change our minds.* He objected that he could hardly change what he hadn't decided. And I reminded him that I was only following through on a plan that *he* had begun before Chance was even dead (the word *traitor* was left unspoken). When the light went on that I was referring to the woman with the beautiful standard poodle, he said, *Not a frou-frou dog, not on your life.* I said I had thought it through carefully. *We won't clip her, she'll look like a long-*

legged lamb that doesn't shed, I said. *What'll we do when we go away?* was his first question. *You've never had a puppy,* I reminded him. *Let's talk about this rationally,* Noel said and sat me down on his knees.

While the West Coast was experiencing its worst snowstorm in seventy-five years, the puppy flew for seventeen hours in the cargo hold of an airplane from Halifax to Vancouver. We sat in the airport playing Scrabble. During our game, a couple passed us towing a crate that held a young Airedale. I kept my regret at ordering a poodle to myself. While we waited past midnight for yet another delayed arrival at an airport unaccustomed to snowstorms, Noel kept assuring me, *She'll be okay – don't worry.* I was sure the puppy would react as neurotically as the ostriches that had got off a plane before hers. They had tried to eat the hair off the men who labored to separate them from their crates.

When the puppy finally arrived, she looked like a lonely little coyote, sleek and clean, her nose pointed and fragile, her eyes curious. Down on my haunches, I began soothing her with the voice that would teach her how to live in trust. As I spoke, I felt two large hands slide between me and the cage door, opening it and reaching in. A look of utter devotion had entered Noel's eyes and he was not looking at me. When he turned toward the door, the puppy was nestled against his neck. *She needs a walk,* he said. In the car, she relaxed on my knee like a rag doll, leaping up at random moments to lick our faces. All semblance of the docile puppy we had first met began to disappear. After an hour the strange little puppy was no longer a stranger, and had in fact brought us all home to each other. A dog's motto seems to be *Give me a place to be, and I'll be there for you.* Where the spirits of human and canine connect, something primal happens.

Too late to catch the ferry back to Victoria, we went to the home of my brother-in-law, Ken, south of Vancouver. Noel and I could not bear to leave the puppy in the van for the night; we felt lonely at the thought of sleeping by ourselves. Having previously phoned Ken to say we would not consider bringing an untrained puppy into his house, we now asked if she could join us. We spent most of the night playing together on the floor. In two hours the puppy had taught us that, indeed, poodles train their owners. They do it the way cats train birds: they toy with them until the ones with access to flight are too exhausted to imagine an escape.

Victoria was too British and common a name for a dog. I named her Chi for life force, but somehow couldn't imagine Noel calling her when she ran off after a seagull. Noel had opted for other names, but I vetoed each of them. Daisy because it had been my mother's name. Second Chance because it had too many syllables to get through when a car barreled down the road. Heidi wouldn't do, either, because it is my chemotherapist's name. Annie was too close to Anne, my second name. Delta would be perfect for a puppy's bladder, but her puppyhood would pass. Finally we decided on Sophia, from the Greek for wisdom. She would provide the wisdom to know the difference between a house without a dog and a home with one. Nothing in her cleverness and energy had shown any semblance of wisdom, but we reasoned that she had many years to prove herself.

When we finally reached home, Sophia met her match. Initially she put a coy paw against her mirror image and licked the tall glass that covers our hall door. Then she began to bound up on all fours, jumping into the air like a lamb. Outraged, she barked at her reflection until the effort threw her back into a sitting position. Surprised, she took a new tack and peered behind the door to catch the enemy off guard. She returned to face the mirror again, then backed away. It appeared to calm her that the intruder in the mirror backed away as well. As she made a tactical rush forward, chaos erupted again. I was reminded of how we rush toward unfounded fears, making them grow large and close, and of how, when we turn away, our demons often recede as well. It is one of the major post-cancer dilemmas – how to learn that our terror of recurrence is often nothing but a reflection of fears that can be avoided by a shift of the gaze or the flexing of muscles.

I flex mine each time we race against Sophia's bladder, bounding toward a place where she feels the wind ruffle her fur and I feel the fresh ocean breeze kiss my lungs. When she deposits something on the grass, I reach to pick it up with a hand covered by a doggie-doo bag. Invariably, she steps on the soft brown pile. Because I am down on her level, she assumes I want to play and jumps up to offer me turd smears and affection. Sometimes an innocent jogger finds herself entangled in Sophia's leash as she leaps out to spread the word of love. Just when I am ready to sell her to the lowest bidder, she sits at the curb unasked and waits for me to tell her she can cross. Sometimes when I reach the other side, she is still waiting, the meaning of *Let's go* having not yet registered. One day at a time, I tell myself, as I used to when I grew discouraged with my treatments.

On one of these days at a time, I came home and marveled at how much more intelligent and sensitive our fourteen-week-old puppy was than some of my colleagues. In two weeks she had acquired some of the wisdom I had hoped for. *Good Sophia,* I said as I looked about for puddles and sniffed the air for worse. She brought me a chewed bit of cardboard to reward my return. *Walk?* I said as I turned into the bedroom. I noticed she backed away, and I noticed too that Noel's newly upholstered chair seemed to glint in the sunlight although the material was a dark, matte blue. A tube of toothpaste sat on the bedroom chair. She had punctured it with the needles that serve for several months as puppy teeth. Sweet mint on smooth cloth had given her something to lick through the leisurely afternoon. Noel learned the story *after* the chair had been scrubbed. Sophia hid behind his long legs as I let rip with my opinion of his suggesting I be *patient*. She cocked her head while I spoke, as though trying to comprehend the unreasonable. Without discussing it, we called her *Sophie* from that night on.

The next day we laughed at my fury and, in a show of generosity, I let Sophie off her leash to experience a moment of freedom. She considered an hour would be preferable and gave us our first lesson in how fast a puppy can run, and how it can wait, head down between its front paws, bum midair, until you've almost got her. Noel tried negotiation, but his aptitude for politics slid past Sophie's apolitical ears. I tried a disciplinary tone that has kept testosterone from overtaking my college classrooms, but my threats set her off toward the busy intersection. Just as a car threatened to mow her down, she dropped her bum onto the curb. When we approached with words of praise, she zipped back onto the boulevard and headed for home. At the gate she waited patiently with something white sticking to the corner of her mouth. As I labored to catch my breath through the scar tissue of my lung, she sat with a cigarette butt clinging to her upper lip. I swear she was smiling.

I have made a few mistakes in my life. I have done things I am ashamed of, said things that caused irreparable damage. I have turned my back on goodness in favor of temporary thrills. I have squandered years on those unworthy of my affection and squandered more time in regret. Some would say, although I believe they oversimplify, that regrets can cause cancer. Nevertheless I regret, with Sophie's arrival, having cut Chance's life shorter than nature would have done. And I have assured Noel that if I live to see Sophie grow old, I will let her choose her own time unless she is in pain. When her bladder is beyond medical science, I will let her sleep winter nights in the warmth of the basement, and summer days in the shade of the apple tree. When she can no longer see or hear, I will be her eyes and ears. When she decides to die, I will rejoice in being alive to bury her.

Germaine Greer wrote that women get older at intervals, that we wake every five years or so to the realization that we look more aged, and finally we become crones. I confess to paying little attention to the slow changes in my appearance. What I have noticed, however, is how the pit of my stomach has aged in its burgeoning sense of vulnerability. After many deaths in my family of blood and friends, after two divorces, and after cancer, I assumed I was no longer able to leap with abandon from past into present. Although I have been trying to live in the moment, I do so with discipline rather than instinct. Sharing love with the right person may still the soul and keep the present tense prominent, but a puppy allows for little beyond the *now*. I cannot agree, however, with those who would rather have dogs than children. I would have preferred my mother's ideal and my grandmother's before her – women who favored having children and *also* a dog for their families to share. A dog is simply a bonus that makes a house more homey, a heart preoccupied.

Hope swells unbidden in the company of Sophie. Tuned to her own immediate needs, she causes our energy to simmer from shared enthusiasm. It comes in the uplift of being forced outside to walk in the untended gardens of nature. All else falls into place during these moments. One of the most treasured things a dog brings its owner is the night sky. When Noel and I walk Sophie before bed, we rediscover what we once had with Chance – the opportunity to gaze at the stars, moon, and with luck, a comet. Away from the traffic, we let Sophie run free along the oceanside.

Sophie is the first puppy who has come to me since I have added the word *mortality* to my vocabulary, and so I sought out godparents. The couple who accepted this office have a chocolate brown poodle – a mischievous male, Bruno, who has spirit enough to understand forty pounds of cream-colored female. I think their duties as godparents may be superfluous, however. Noel is experiencing his first puppy. He finds her staring into his face when he wakes in the morning, her chin propped on the edge of the bed. Her uninhibited joy when he comes home from bureaucratic bafflegab never wanes. I have heard him apologize to her that he could not show the same exuberance as she does when he opens the door at the end of the day. In exchange for her place to be, Sophie has created for us a language without a glimmer of sorrow.

People say Noel is a man of restraint; Sophie and I know differently. I have tried to warn him that one grows grateful for even the smallest acts of obedience in a young dog, the simplest signs of love, and then suddenly the dog is perfectly in tune, and just as suddenly she is old beyond playfulness. I shared with him the thought that if we should have the good fortune to see Sophie into her dotage, we would never have her put to sleep. Our next puppy would simply have to adjust to the three of us as we grew old together. *Our next puppy?* he asked, looking a bit tired as he searched for a leather glove last seen leaving the room in Sophie's mouth. But my husband, to his own surprise, has proven himself a pushover for the love that lives at his own address.

❧ 11 ❧

Spirit Cleansers

Dina has cleaned my house every second Thursday since 1983. At least once a year she reminds me that she intends to retire to her homeland, just to make sure that I appreciate her. Having moved with her husband from the Azores almost twenty years ago, Dina has raised four children in Canada, bought herself a four-wheel drive, and planted a massive garden around her house, but she has not passed her driving test. Ironically this woman who cleans houses for several members of an English department is unable to read or write English. Perhaps we conspire against her because she has confessed she will return to the house she still owns in Portugal as soon as she can take a driver's license with her.

I discovered Dina was illiterate when she disappeared unexpectedly and I replaced her with a woman from Vietnam. Six weeks later Dina called to say she would be back the following Thursday. She reacted like a jealous lover when I told her I had hired someone else to clean my house. I suspect she thought I would appreciate her more if I had to do the work myself or sleep over the slut's wool that gathers under the bed. *I come back*, she told me in a tone that suggested I fire the other woman or else. When she arrived I tried to make clear who was the mistress of the house. *You didn't tell me, Dina. I was surprised when I came home to a mess*, I explained. *I tell*, she said, pointing to the calendar on our kitchen door: *I make X*. And so she had. There under every second Thursday were tiny X's to mark her trip back to the Azores.

Years before cancer entered my life, I hired Dina on the advice of a member of my department; she eventually made the rounds to work in the homes of five others. We were then privy to one another's dirt, literal and metaphoric. I, for example, met Dina at a difficult time in my life. My mother had been hospitalized that fall, and I was trying to keep order in my father's home and my own, as well as dealing with my students' essays and my lectures. I ferried back and forth on weekends from Victoria to the mainland, growing steadily more tired with the despair of Mother's struggle and the upkeep of two houses. The year after my sisters and I helped our father bury our mother, Lynne found him his own cleaning woman. He referred to her as *a stranger in my house* until he surprised himself by sitting down to tea with her.

When my father died, my second husband took the approach, as he had when Mother died, that death was an inconvenience, especially if it fell just before a Halloween party. After all, a funeral lasts only a couple of hours, so why was I so glum the following weekend? Other women were apparently ready to entertain husbands whose wives needed to mourn the loss of a parent. There seemed no point in two people being sad under the same roof if one could avoid it.

Dina continued to keep my house in order during my divorce. She remained constant too when my older sister began her slow descent. Yellow rubber gloves flashing as she emphasized her point, Dina advised me about my *he-bad* ex-husband, my *she-no-like* arthritic dog, Chance, and the *you-color* silver that had begun to thread itself through my dark brown hair. I had always thought my sprinkling of silver hair made me look sophisticated, but my second husband and Dina had both been bent on teaching me that bleach keeps the sheets messy with sex when it's not being used to keep them white. I consoled myself with comments about *real* men, but neither of them paid any attention. My second husband went off with a middle-aged dye job, and Dina told me to ponder the wisdom of my rival: *She know he like.* In fact Dina seemed to feel that the whole neighborhood might support her view if she let them know her opinion. As I put my briefcase into the car one day, she yelled across the lawn from the top of my front steps, waving my old T-shirt that she used for a cleaning cloth: *You color, like me. You look young then.* I waved good-bye while she stood clenching a swath of her own blackened hair in a yellow-gloved hand to point out how I would look.

Though in her late fifties and less than five feet tall, Dina is formidable, and I have always been slightly afraid of her. She seldom speaks at normal volume, shouting from the moment she bursts through the door until she leaves. Neither are her opinions limited to laundry detergents and cleaning tools. After her first year of working for me, she poked me in the stomach one morning as we passed in the hall: *Why you have no baby? You too skinny?* There are few things I like to hear more than suggestions that I am underweight but even this comment did not lessen my upset. She covered the silence by describing her children and grandchildren. *I bring pictures,* she shouted, as though to encourage me to reconsider parenting.

But Dina and I had our longest argument over a mop. *This will mean you don't have to be down on your knees all morning,* I said, passing her the new mop with its levered handle to squeeze the attached sponge without bending. She looked about as grateful as she did the day I put skim milk in her coffee. *It blue,* she said, informing me that she *drink milk.* When I returned home from work the day I gave her the mop, I found it in the basement. *Use it!* I encouraged the next time she burst into my solitude. *It will be easier for your back and knees.* I felt guilty sitting in a chair marking papers while she was on her knees scrubbing away my dirt. As always she won by endurance and volume. I would come home to find the vases full of flowers and the mop hidden in some distant part of the basement.

Dina has opinions about most things, but her favorite topic is men and her control over them. She had tried to tell me about my second husband: *He not like you.* She may have meant he and I were not alike, or perhaps that she had realized before I did that he no longer liked me. I never had a chance to ask because she launched into a tirade about her sister's husband, who beat his wife. *He stupid man.* Against my better judgment, I asked why her sister had not broken off with him. *No good woman leave man,* Dina advised me. I was left to wonder whether there was no advantage in leaving a man or whether only a bad woman left her man. *You no live lone,* she added, which I interpreted to mean that alone I was not a good woman, although I could not imagine how I could get into trouble with a man when I did not have one around.

Dina met Noel before he became my husband. He was visiting me in hospital when I was having my first biopsy. As he and I said good-bye at the elevator door, she appeared with her flushed Portuguese husband, who always came with a small black dog to pick her up. This day he wore a green hospital gown; Dina had his trousers draped over her arm. Feeling some need to explain my own gown, I told her I had a terrible cough and it might be pneumonia. *You wear socks,* she said in a voice that could wake the geriatric ward. Then she made a surreptitious and throaty guffaw while she told us why she was carrying her husband's trousers. *I take home pants so he no come home.* With a surge of pride, she said that if she left his clothes or any money with him, he would dress himself and follow her home on the bus. More surprising was the reason for his escapes: *He need me talk doctors.* Apparently she translated for him, taking the doctors to task if their medicines had a foul taste or her husband's stomach pains persisted. Like me, her husband stood by in trepidation.

When Noel moved into the house, Dina said, *I know man here. I see shoes.* She grinned and waited for me to explain the lascivious details, perhaps to enlighten my colleagues. When I disappointed her, she followed me to my study with suggestions that I learn to make sweet breads and grow my own grapes to make special wines. *I teach,* she offered. When Noel and I married, she said, *You lucky girl!* I wanted to ask why she didn't think he was lucky too, but feared the answer.

Sometimes things were a bit tricky between Dina and Chance, who in her old age did not like to be told to move. Usually Chance's dimmed hearing barely registered Dina's order when the dog's corner of my study was invaded by the roaring vacuum. *She no like,* Dina complained when Chance growled or stayed put. *I teach,* she told me, as though I were remiss in discipline as well as fertility. But Dina and Chance were a match in stubbornness. I left them to quarrel it out, having learned that they had enough fear of each other to keep their arguments short of physical violence.

After Sophie came into our lives and the floors grew cluttered and scuffed, Dina began advising me about how to raise her: *She no listen you. She listen me.* As she spoke she glanced at the glass door with its muddy smudges and scratched frame. *I say, she do.* Sophie proved Dina true. She greeted her with abandon and then followed her around like a German shepherd trained by the police force. *How do you do it?* I asked, genuinely curious. Dina dragged a rug half her weight to the deck to beat it into submission, and the puppy followed her outside. *She listen me,* Dina answered as Sophie sat waiting for her next command. It occurred to me that perhaps dogs do indeed behave just like their owners.

Dina has been in charge for almost a decade and a half while I hide out in my study or at the college. I have learned over the years to shout back when she barges into my study or complains about my choice of cleansers or corrects the pronunciation of a friend who is teaching me Italian. She and I both act on the premise that were we to speak at normal volume, the earth would slow to a crawl, as it did one morning in March of 1995.

On this day, I was bedded down for the supremely humbling experience of my first chemotherapy treatment. Having ignored until too late the ten glasses of water that must accompany an injection, I had become frail, dehydrated, and discouraged. Try as I might, I could not lift my head from the pillow, and my tongue felt like someone had stuffed an angora mitten in my mouth. I was also at that stage when I feared if I owned up to having cancer, it might stick around and my new love might not. And so Dina found me when she arrived to tear the sheets from under the quilt. *You bed!* she scolded me, hands on her tiny hips. *I'm sorry, Dina,* I began, and the tears that she had not seen over other partings now slipped down my face and onto the pillow as we contemplated the fact that I was not about to leap out of bed. *You sick?* she asked. *Oh well,* I told her, wondering why I was brave in front of doctors and colleagues but a disaster in front of my cleaning woman. *The doctors say I have cancer.*

Dina thought for a moment in the only silence we have ever shared while occupying the same room. She bent her head and looked lost for an opinion for the first time. When she raised her eyes they were full of tears. *You sick head?* she asked in a hushed voice, having always been of the opinion that I knew more about books than men. I shook my head. *In my chest,* I answered, hand over my heart, pulling down the cover a bit to show her where my scar began. *No Elizabat! You no cancer,* she whispered. *You smile, you better.* Having learned to interpret her, I knew she was not commanding me to smile, but rather suggesting that I would get better if I managed to change my sorrowful face to a happy one. *I no leave, you smile,* she said, which can loosely be translated to mean that if I didn't wipe the downcast look off my face, she would stand there all day, arms akimbo, and I would have to clean the house myself.

My bulbous tongue, fluttering heart, and newly stitched chest argued against the inclination, but I began to laugh. Dina looked as though she had just salvaged the western hemisphere from nuclear attack. Her gloved hands left her hips to dangle by her sides, free at last. *You no smile, you no live,* she said. *I fix; I make sweet bread.* Imagining something heavy and sweet as it maneuvered past my swollen tongue, I felt my throat close. *You like,* she said. And she left the room to battle with Chance and bang about in the kitchen.

In the lulling discord of her caring, I slipped into a momentary sleep but was awakened when the basement door slammed. Dina returned to my bedroom. *I mop,* she said, holding in her hand the instrument of our ancient quarrel. I slept the rest of the morning, dreaming of mountain streams whose rivulets drained into the desert of my flesh.

Just as Dina taught me about the wellsprings of comfort, other females have taught me that a family of friends can soothe the absence of kindred blood. On our last Christmas together, my mother had asked me to convince my father of the futility of loyalty beyond the grave. I knew she could not bear the thought of his being alone for the rest of his life, and she knew he would have choices. He refused to discuss the idea of settling into a new life once she had passed out of ours. After she died, I was unable to encourage him to widen his horizons, in spite of the eager support of various retired women. He died missing Mother as much as he had at the beginning of his loss. My mother's wish for his happiness and my father's overwhelming loneliness inadvertently taught me to widen my horizons after my cancer diagnosis.

In the same way I had learned to trust in the love of another man and to rejoice in the company of another dog, I began to fill the void left by my sisters – one dead, the other estranged – with the companionship of cherished friends. When Noel and I married, many of our middle-aged friends and relatives arrived at the ceremony with silvering temples and compact cameras. Perhaps because they seldom attend weddings of members of their own generation, or perhaps in response to our decision to have no formal photographs, guests later sent us some nine hundred shots of the celebration. Having survived cancer for over a year, I was not certain I could survive organizing this amazing stack of pictures. I asked twenty-four female friends to join me in sorting and scissoring the snapshots into collages now bound together in a beautiful album. As I served punch and biscotti to my guests, I realized that although the photographs include both my brothers-in-law, neither of my sisters had come to rest between the album covers.

I knew before the wedding that neither sister would be there, of course, but facts seldom comfort the soul. No one replaces a sister, although bountiful friendships make the absence less painful. The problem is that my family of friends had not been there when I was in the process of *becoming*. Divorce had compounded this emptiness for me because Noel had had no chance to know my parents or sisters, as my two former husbands had. Although my previous husbands have little in common besides having been married to me, they both gravitated toward my family. I have no earthly continuum with this family now, nor is there reason to expect the one Margaret Mead promised sisters in their post-menopausal years — a time, she said, when sisters grow to enjoy the strongest relationship.

My sisters' faces, their high cheekbones and lovely eyes — Joyce's warm chocolate, Lynne's summer blue — remind me of all that can transpire to change the face of family. And as each friend snipped the photographed faces to glue on her collage, I felt an absence that *knowing* cannot mend. Rare as perfection is in families, there seems a persistent desire among women to live within the white picket fence of sisterly love. The flower of this relationship roots itself in different soil than friendship does. As the petals of sisterhood dry and fall, they bring with them a message about the end of something essential and reflect a former self that a woman may wish simultaneously to escape and to embrace.

Friends gain access to us through common interests rather than common parents. The intimacy of friendship allows us to feel safe in knowing that we can gentle ourselves away from its excesses, in contrast to sisters who remain rooted to a permanent place if they are there for us at all. Perhaps, too, we can more easily absorb important lessons through the lives of our friends because their failures and triumphs do not reflect on our pride in the way that a sister's does. Neither are those ingrained habits of family around to push the wrong buttons and create knee-jerk responses. It is both a strength and a weakness that the bonds of sisterhood thwart our ability to change.

The major conduit that differentiates friends and sisters is obviously the one that carries our blood to and from our hearts. And perhaps it is this very heart-of-family that most compels us to maintain some link, however tenuous. Carol Shields reflects on this genetic print in her poem "Sister." Using the image of an identical wrist, she describes how a familial gesture links her to both her sister and her dead mother, *reminding us/exactly who she was,/who we are.* I am reminded how often people have guessed that Lynne and I are related because of something in our faces and in the way we mimick each other in our expressions. I remember too the physical similarities that my newly widowed father pointed out as he dried the dishes while I washed them: *You have your mother's hands,* he said in a voice tinged with love and loss. It occurred to me then that I would recognize my sisters' hands anywhere and that I can conjure them up at whim. The connection of flesh and blood creates a unique and indelible tattoo on our *being.* Perhaps this is why we long to escape it while at the same time we cannot help but be profoundly moved by those who were bred by the same bones.

When my friends had finished their collages and begun to clean up paper scraps, I asked them about their own sisters. Perhaps I was looking for vicarious joy or company in sorrow, but I was amazed by their reactions. Each woman conveyed intensely complex emotions. With a few exceptions, their responses fit into three categories. First there were those whose parents had divorced or divided before the children had left home, a much less publicized phenomenon during the 1940s, fifties, and early sixties than it is today. As a consequence the siblings had grown up inextricably bound to one another in youthful self-defense. Second were those who lived so far from siblings that visits were yearly at best, and hence they were not subjected to the frequent visits that can wear out a sibling's welcome and open the door on old differences and new quarrels. Love renews itself in intermittent absence. And third were those who grew up to discover that their sisters were people with whom they had little in common beyond the habit of calling the same people their parents. Still, when my friends spoke of their siblings, even in anger or seeming indifference, I sensed a longing for resolution, a yearning as though for something intangible now lost. Intermingled with these wistful complaints, I heard repeatedly each woman's need to exonerate herself in ways she would never feel compelled to do with friends: *I love my sister; it's just that....*

Perhaps the most heart-warming story I heard came from Noel's family. When I married Noel, I gained a mother-in-law, Lily, and an extended family that includes my mother-in-law's sister, Claire. Lily and Claire are less than a year apart in age. As I write, my mother-in-law is within weeks of her ninetieth birthday. Both women have been widowed for years from the men they still love. Their empty nests allow them to live together for six months in Victoria and then to separate for summer and autumn, when Lily returns to her apartment in Winnipeg. Like Lynne and me, Lily and Claire lost a sister to cancer; they too carry her face and expressions.

I mentioned to these elderly sisters how lucky they were to each have a home with two bedrooms so that they could be together without crowding. They looked astonished and said they had never spent a night apart under the same roof. *We always sleep in the same bed, just like we did on the farm*, Lily told me. Claire explained that they could talk into the night this way, and then she confessed, *I'm a reader and she's not.* My new mother-in-law agreed, telling me she enjoyed her sister's shortened version of each novel because *I've always been the impatient one.* As they spoke, each gave the other credit for their lasting affections, and when they finished talking of each other they talked about their eldest sister in Vancouver. To their surprise, this eldest sister is beginning to feel her age at ninety-three. *She lost her son – only twenty, you know,* they told me, as if this tragedy in early middle age explained why she had to have a hip replacement in her nineties. These sisters made me realize that, even without the ravages of cancer, life is too short to waste in silence. Why couldn't Lynne and I age like Lily and Claire, or sing our way through the years like Kate and Anna McGarrigle?

Perhaps the answer begins with our elder sister. Joyce disapproved when Lynne or I did anything differently from her. Most painful for me was her refusal to accept my not having children. The fact that I adored her five babies and had been through the Harvard Medical Clinic and several Canadian institutions in an effort to find the cause of my barrenness left no impression on her. Stubbornly, she believed that the pleasure I found in my career negated the possibility that I could enjoy motherhood. Her inflexible views on parenting and a woman's place encouraged me to be cautious about what I shared with her. And like the next domino poised to fall, I took the same stance of superior wisdom over

Lynne, causing her to manipulate, astonish, or avoid me when her infatuation with encounter groups or exaggerated stories failed to stimulate my appetite. In combination, we all contributed to the tumbling down of our affections. This tradition continued into our early middle age, when our birth order was no longer so physically apparent. These habits were no longer relevant or desirable, but simply and irresistibly entrenched.

I see now that Joyce felt trapped at home sometimes, while Lynne and I traveled and went to university. In return, I saw her as a woman fulfilled by motherhood while I lived in hope from month to month. I see too that Lynne has come late in life to the need to take responsibility for herself, to resist making herself the center of attention. She does not want to be accountable as long as there are others around to blame, or to impress with her woes, but how could she be otherwise as the youngest by so many years? My position as the middle child afforded me the luxury of sharing some understanding with both sisters that they could not share with each other.

Joyce was born late in the second year of my parents' marriage, before my father had adapted to the idea that he would have to share my mother with anyone else. She had to fulfill the impossible expectations that come with being first born, and she raged against my mother's notions of control. She also softened the crib for me. I was born six years later to a father who not only wanted another child, but who said I reminded him of his own mother. Lynne, who followed six years after me, was the daughter of parents who had not expected more children. She was a surprise to my father and a source of pride to a mother in her late thirties. As a teen-ager, Lynne became the one through whom my mother could find her youth again.

As T.S. Eliot wrote, *in the end we return to the beginning to see the place for the first time.* I realize now how different the context of each sister's birth family was, ranging from the Depression years of the mid-thirties, to the wartime years of the early forties, to the prosperity at the end of that decade. The difficulty we three sisters had in sustaining an intimate bond was fostered by real differences. The year Joyce was watching her breasts develop and feeling fearful of having to ask for a sanitary pad, Lynne was dirtying her diapers and sucking nourishment from our mother's breasts. Caught between them, I wished I could be breast-fed and grown-up at the same time.

Money – the lack of it or the privileges it buys – is often the source of change in families. It affects the pride girls feel as they grow up. Before Lynne was born, my grandparents moved into our small white house in Winnipeg. Mother was able to work outside the home to help with wartime wages while my maternal grandmother lifted me out of the crib and sent Joyce off to school. My parents put my crib in their room and my grandparents in the second bedroom. At the age of eight, Joyce spent each night on two separate beds. She slept in my parents' bed until it was bedtime for the adults. Then my father would carry her to the living-room couch where my mother covered her in blankets. She woke each morning with a household of traffic moving toward the bathroom, the breakfast table, and the front door. How could she have developed the same values as her younger sisters? I had the privacy of my own bed at thirteen, when Joyce married, and Lynne had the luxury of an entire bedroom when she became a teen-ager. Joyce was the forerunner who had no chance to carve out a space for herself before the first of her children came into the world. She carried the weight of her parents' learning process into her own.

There were happy times with my sisters, of course. Two stand out as precious moments of spontaneous affection. Lynne decided at age twenty-two to work in Germany. At the peak of her nubile beauty, she needed to escape the watchful eye of our mother. I was at a turning point in my own life and bought an airplane ticket to Heidelberg to join her for a train ride to Greece. When I arrived, we had barely begun talking when she leapt off her bed and threw her arms around me, telling me with uncharacteristic exuberance how happy she was to be together again. Perhaps she was remembering the times I had left our childhood kitchen with my shoes full of the bread crusts she refused to eat and wanted to hide from our mother. Her welcome warms me even now, a quarter century later.

Similarly Joyce surprised me. She had made no secret of her disapproval of divorce, and in particular of my leaving my first husband to go to university, an exchange of sorrow for enlightenment. She even disapproved of my divorcing my second husband, despite his repeated unfaithfulness. Years later, though, as she lay dying, she burst out with enthusiasm for my life as a newly single woman: *What do you need him for anyway?* she asked. *You can be happy on your own!* I had to turn away to hide the depth of gratitude I felt. From that moment on our pasts melted away, and for the next four months I became *her* nurturing big sister. When she moved closer to death, her face shone each time I came to her bedside. She died having taught me that as long as there is life, a change of heart is possible.

With Joyce's death, our original family of five was whittled down to two. Except for my parents' and sister's funerals, or when I visited Lynne's ex-husband for my annual dental work, I had seldom seen her in a decade. We lived no more than four hours' travel from each other, but she had stopped calling or returning my calls. If I tried to discuss the problem she would end the conversation by saying that someone was at her door or that supper was burning. I was grateful and surprised, then, by her visits during my initial cancer treatments. In a semi-conscious state of grief, I phoned her and she took the ferry from the mainland to Victoria, bringing with her a dozen pink roses that I later dried. When I was well enough to turn onto my stomach, she came with yellow roses and gave me a massage while her youngest son played his guitar.

On her third visit I took a deep breath during the massage and asked why, after our wonderful travels in the sixties and visits in the seventies, she had suddenly shut me out of her life. I confessed I was afraid for myself with my terminal diagnosis, and for her now that she was headed down the lonely road toward divorce and self-reliance. I knew when I felt her hands freeze that I should have remained content within the present gift of renewed sisterhood. She told me she *must have had a reason* for her sudden distance, and never visited me again.

When my cancer went into remission and Noel and I decided to marry, I sent Lynne a letter asking her to take part in the ceremony. Without explanation she refused, returning her invitation with *Regrets* penned in the margin. In need of some semblance of normalcy in the face of Noel's extended family, I gathered the precious remnants of my own family around me. My elder brother-in-law, Bob, brought his daughter, Angela, and her new husband; my younger brother-in-law, Ken, gave me away; and Lynne and Ken's son, Jordan, served the wedding cake.

I may have offended Lynne by asking her former husband to play a role in the ceremony, in spite of his quarter century of undemonstrative but loyal friendship with me. I had, however, invited her to perform on the grand piano if she wished or to bring her younger son, Luke, and mingle with the guests. I assume she wanted Noel and me to make her marital quarrel our own, although she had never denied herself the freedom to see either of my past husbands when the opportunity arose. She wasn't there to see her elder son serve the wedding cake along with Joyce's daughter and my stepdaughter, Camille. She wasn't there to be photographed with Noel's family. I try not to ponder too long or too often how I could have nipped our problem in the bud of its malforming. But when, on occasion, I awaken with a heavy heart, I see my sister's face and feel diminished by her absence.

Years ago Lynne gave me two healing crystals, as though she knew that some day I would need them. They catch the sunshine from my windows now, casting their rainbows as they dance on the walls. They remind me that although she and I lost our affection in the disorder of change, I have not yet given up hope that there is still an *us* somewhere. But over the years, I have come to depend on the robust blessings of my female friends. These women have been my strength when I had none, my beacons when I was lost, and my support on my wedding day – a sisterhood.

Recently, when many of these friends created my wedding collages, we inadvertently left the final page of the album blank. It gives me comfort in my remission to see there is a space to fill, special days yet to come, candles to blow out and relight. Perhaps one day my sister will share in a celebration with me, and I will have a photograph to paste into my album. In the golden light of the moment, dreams are still important.

In the meantime, Dina comes every second Thursday to clean my house and give me advice. She yells and mops and bangs about. And she dusts the crystals Lynne gave me, so they will continue to turn sunlight into rainbows.

✤ 12 ✤

Garden of the Soul

Writing a book had not entered my imagination when I began scribbling my way toward wellness, but the process has become one of my survival strategies. Even when I am too vulnerable or too exuberant to write objectively, I can achieve perspective by refining my thoughts. After years of teaching Canadian literature, I realize that the writer makes half the story and the reader creates the other half. The making of a book became my way of reaching beyond the limits of my surroundings, connecting to that other half.

During my radiation and chemotherapy treatments, I began my days as I had for many years. I read the *Globe and Mail* while I ate a bagel and drank tea. One morning I decided to say something back to the paper and wrote a brief satire. My effort, "Love, Support, and Other Intrusions," was meant to communicate that family and friends mean a great deal to a confused and fearful cancer patient, that their kindness heals the spirit.

Months later, as I read my words in national newsprint at a ski lodge in Whistler, it seemed my life was unfolding as I had always hoped. Two words turned me from rapture to remorse: *Crabbiness appropriate.* I shook my fist at the gods and asked what they had done with my verb. I tried to reason that through imperfection we learn to recognize perfection, should it ever pass our way. *A sentence fragment*, I whispered to Noel, as though the ears of the world were upon us. *No one's going to notice*, he consoled. *My colleagues will*, I told him. Cancer seemed less shameful than an English instructor with a sentence fragment attached to her name in the national news. Noel reminded me that I had other plans for the day. Before the paper had arrived, we had been wondering if my lungs could withstand the combination of altitude and cold on the slopes, and he suggested it was time to find out. As he talked me into my ski suit, I wondered who at the *Globe* hated me.

But Noel was right. Either no one noticed the error or those I spoke with were too generous to mention it. What did happen, however, astonished me. In the days to follow I learned that some readers had thought my piece ungrateful and hardhearted. When they read my suggestion, for example, that caregivers put cooking instructions on their casseroles before they leave pots on my doorstep or that people not disturb me when I was blissed out on morphine, they were offended. Perhaps satire was not within everyone's reach first thing in the morning.

I wrote another article, "The Perfection of Hope," and popped it in the mailbox with a letter to the *Globe* asking the editor if I could polish a short piece about any of the cancer treatments I discussed. To my astonishment, she accepted the entire draft, and I was offered the delicious task of refining the piece for an entire page in the Saturday edition. My life was brim full as I discovered that writing, for all its bum-numbing reality, is a stimulating and satisfying pastime, complete unto itself. The more I wrote, the less I felt like a helpless victim afloat on a sea of cancer cells. I imagined myself, instead, swimming down a river of words that simply needed netting to convey the message of hope.

The *Globe* was sending a photographer for a picture to go with my article. Each morning for three days I sat on my doorstep with my hair washed, but no one came. When the photographer finally arrived, she was young enough to be my daughter. Whatever she bade me do I did several times over for the various angles of her lens. When she asked me to jump over Father Sweeney's grave in the Ross Bay Cemetery, I bounded over his ancient tomb, my lace-up boots and shawl airborne with my spirit. Later, huffing and puffing, I reached home and, with my boots still on, fell asleep near the front door.

The gods of the afterlife had been watching my grave-jumping sacrilege. When I awoke, my torso burned with a deep itching. When I scratched, it felt as though someone were scraping at my nerve endings with a hat pin. In the mirror, a necklace of red welts stared back at me. At a walk-in clinic, I was diagnosed as having shingles, a common low-immunity response in patients who have recently finished cancer treatments. My resistance had collapsed in the face of a virus lying dormant in my body.

The article on hope landed with a familiar slap on my doorstep one Saturday in March. I was unprepared for the response. A flood of phone calls and letters from readers made me realize how many people are interested in combining complementary therapies with conventional ones. Some had been told by skeptics that health benefits gained during alternative therapies were simply a product of chance or just a matter of comfort. I understand the word *comfort*, but I do not understand the word *just*. It's analogous to a man's telling his wife that his affair was *just sex*. Comfort, like sex, is what people want as part of the package. There's no *just* about it.

At first I felt a bit fraudulent talking to people about cancer because I knew so little about its enormous complexities; eventually I reasoned that the medical profession was having the same problem, and so I carried on. Patients simply needed to share their experiences after being tattooed with exhausting rays and dehydrating needles. Bruce Cockburn sings about a universal need for the milk of human kindness to combat a disease that does not distinguish the banker's desk from the derelict's fire: *in the absence of compassion there is cancer/whose banner flies over palaces and mean streets.* Oncologists have little time to spend in discussion as the line-up of patients grows steadily longer; neither have they time to risk on emotional connections. With medical scientists still seeking a cancer cure, the oncologist has to move into the fray with nerves steady and courage intact. Patients soon realize that the breath of life through which we connect with the living world is dependent on more than medicines. As yoga teaches, it also depends on the ephemeral balance between our inner and outer worlds.

Most patients tend to do a form of research-on-the-run and wish to share their findings with those who understand fear and loneliness. One story between patients is worth a library of statistics, especially since statistics usually deal with losses instead of gains. I wonder, for example, why statistics on lung cancer published in early 1997 begin by saying that 80 percent of patients will die within five years. I would prefer to read that 20 percent of lung cancer patients, an entire fifth of those afflicted, will be swilling their vegetable soup at the end of five years. Cancer patients need a motive for sleeping at night and for climbing out of bed in the morning. They need a reason to move forward into something other than death.

The response to my essay confirmed the basic premise of

alternative therapies: to be well, one must seek balance through nurturing the whole self. I have learned that most doctors, if drawn into conversation, express a belief that the body cannot thrive if the spirit is not willing. Doctors call it *attitude*. Initially I needed help with my attitude. When I had absorbed the reality of my circumstances, I felt low-down and mean about the costly misdiagnoses that had scarred my body inside and out. I needed to let that feeling go.

Now, after two years of regular medical monitoring and weekly alternative therapies, I seldom allow my moods to go slumming. When acupuncture frees up the energy flow along my meridians and massage soothes the savage twins of fear and tension, I carry the threat of metastasis in a smaller pocket than otherwise. When naturopathy prods my immune system and yoga gathers my energies into a balanced force, I can allow my reach to exceed my grasp again. When I use their combined sustenance to stir my creative juices, it seems that cancer has the potential to be – oddly enough – a blessing.

I am reminded of my friend Jane, who says, *Depression is the luxury of the idle.* She means that we have to be productive to be happy. I agree with her, but remission requires the discipline of calm as well. Sometimes my brain idles when I overextend myself. I shuddered with embarrassment after I had bought the lamb's wool coat of my dreams to wear to a conference. When I brought the coat home and slipped it on to model for Noel, we discovered a stain inside the lapel. I realized that I had not adequately registered the price tag, which had *as is* written beside the sale price. The store owner was generous, however, and agreed to have a monogram of my initials embroidered over the stain. Before leaving for my flight, I rushed into the store and asked to see my *mammogram* instead of my monogram. We laughed at the slip of my tongue, but

I recognized how cancer pushes forward when the mind is idle. It takes a certain alertness to keep dread from taking over.

Sometimes too it is hard to dissipate the anger that accompanies hopelessness. I felt bile rise when I listened to a doctor lecturing the public on the power of the patient. She used a navigational metaphor, likening the patient to the captain of a ship. The problem with this metaphor is that it doesn't work. Metaphors are supposed to clarify things, but this one would confuse any person who has been seriously ill and mislead anyone who has not. The captain of a ship acquires his job because he is seen to deserve it. Few people deserve their illnesses. The captain deserves his position because he knows everything about his ship. The patient knows little about her own ship when cancer strikes. Broccoli, carrots, and meditation may assist prevention and help to maintain remissions, but they cannot be expected to cure a serious disease. In fact, doctors seldom eradicate cancer without surgeries that require further doctors to anesthetize, cut, sew, and medicate patients.

A captain has supreme power over those afloat with him and he has access to all the ship's equipment. All egos are sublimated to his authority, enabling him to move forward as a benevolent dictator. This posture seldom works between doctor and patient because the patient runs smack up against the doctor's ego. As well, the captain must be alert, fit, and knowledgable. A patient – tired, fearful, and confused – seldom has the knowledge to run the medical equipment necessary for survival. After a life-changing diagnosis and the harshness of conventional treatments, patients feel fragile and dependent. We go to our doctors in the hope they can sail us through the storm of our afflictions, not so we can skipper a ship that has become frightening and unfamiliar. The cliché about the captain going down with the ship is the only part that rings metaphorically true.

This doctor also spoke about the patient's power to hire and fire doctors. In most Canadian cities, the number of doctors per patient is lessening, and the difficulty of getting in to see a good doctor is increasing. In Victoria, a doctor without a waiting list is a doctor to beware. Entering a reputable doctor's office takes both pull and push. The door was opened for me by a friend who is married to a specialist and who came to stay with me on a visit home from Saudi Arabia. She got me into the office of another of her friends, one of the best general practitioners in Victoria. After being misdiagnosed, I needed this new doctor to restore my confidence. Neither could I visit a specialist or have any tests done without this doctor's blessing. While my cancer spread, my first general practitioner had stood between me and the x-ray machine in spite of my bloody sputum and exhaustion. In time, I had to work my resentment out with meditation, exercise, and the counsel of friends: *Why waste today's thoughts on yesterday's problems?* My current doctors are supportive and generous in their energies and time. But my being able to visit them has nothing to do with my authority to hire and fire; it has to do with friendship and happenstance.

Between calls prompted by my article about hope, I sat at my computer to do what I had always done when I needed grounding. I wrote stories that linked the lessons of my life together, and stuffed the pages into file folders. During one of these moments, the phone rang again. I was suspicious and hesitant when the male voice on the other end introduced himself as a publisher who had read my essay. He then asked a question that would not compute at first because I had known too much sorrow. He asked if he could publish my book. Perhaps I should have been more confident because my divorce lawyer had responded to my correspondence in the late 1980s by suggesting I write a book about the experience of divorce. She said that women needed to know how to keep some humor and steadiness throughout the ordeal. Once the legal papers made me single again, however, I gave a great sigh and stuffed the story of divorce into a file.

Something about cancer made me want to reach out. Perhaps it is the profound loneliness of being part of a group no one wants to join. I thought about the publisher's offer for a long six seconds before excitement began to rise from my toes. If a publisher was willing to print my stories, all I had to do was stay well enough to write them. *What makes you think I've got a book in me?* I asked. He explained that he knew something about the business of putting books on bookstore shelves, and that he had put a few of his own books there as well. In my excitement I forgot what he said as quickly as he said it, but I was sufficiently impressed to wonder if he had called the wrong number. Before he could consider this possibility too, I agreed, especially as he said I could use my original title on the book. When we hung up, I phoned a local bookseller as well as my *Globe* editor to make certain the publisher was for real. Both assured me I should sit down and write.

From the moment I said *yes*, I began to solidify my sense of cancer as an opportunity rather than an affliction. Once I had joined forces with the disease, I felt less fearful about the illness and more fearful about finding the right words to express what I had learned. With a little help from my friends, I have been able to turn cancer from an end to a beginning. Whether I live a long life or not, I will rest between the covers of my book, sitting on the shelves of people known and unknown to me, keeping them company. The power of a stranger's invitation has allowed me to write my way into a community of light.

This transformation beckoned me to look on my cancer with perspective. *Reculer pour mieux sauter,* say the French, step back and wait for the opportunity to leap farther forward with renewed energy. Although I have had to meet the physical and emotional pain of cancer, I have tried to step back and acknowledge my stress and reply to it with tenderness and truth. I befriend myself by circling the dark shadows of my mind and accommodating them by whatever means I can. These means more often than not involve the generosity of others, and the discipline of putting pen to paper.

A silly expression bounced into my thoughts one day when I was shaky with exhaustion and yet wanting to finish one more paragraph, talk to one more student, and fold one more load of laundry: *pruning power.* The words made me laugh. In pondering them, I realized my problem. The clarity of thought that allows me to make good choices is absent when I grow tired, but instead of resting I become driven to finish what I am doing. On bad days, the more tired I get, the more I clutch to my chore, temper blazing when someone tries to slow me down. Fortunately I married a patient man who does not take other people's flaws personally, especially his wife's. With a few well-chosen phrases, he convinces me that I would work more efficiently if I napped and ate at regular intervals. He also persuades me that I should nap in silence and eat in company. The taped books I bought to entertain myself when I rested have been replaced with meditative breathing; the print-outs I used to bring to the table remain in my study. Unbidden, Sophie has decided to rest with me during nap time and to sit under my chair as I eat. In sly cooperation with my husband, she steadies me into the moment.

The noun *prune* makes me think of the partially dried fruit from the plum tree of years ago in my parents' backyard, the medicine my mother encouraged us to take when we were constipated. Sometimes she served prunes for breakfast or for dessert and we realized she was trying to make us let go, get on with our day. We weren't allowed to talk about our bowels at the table or in polite company. Even in private we numbered our bathroom activities. In the medical world, of course, these unmentionables are a source of lengthy discussion and an excellent diagnostic tool. They assist us in knowing when our bodies are not working properly to wash away toxic visitors.

The verb *to prune* I learned from my mother as well. An avid gardener, she believed in pruning off the dead bits that encumbered her plants or trees. At some point, she taught me that pruning allows the life force to flourish. For me, *pruning power* sums up the notion of relieving myself of physical and spiritual toxins, and lopping off dead issues to blossom anew.

Since my stint in the clinic my body has not worked as well as it once did, although it works much better than it did in the months of coughing, prior to radiation and chemotherapy. But no matter how much rest and good fortune come my way, I am physically weakened. If I acknowledge these limitations, I filter out disappointment. Often my mind and spirit have to nudge my body along. At other times, I become fed up with my decreased stamina and my fearful caution. Although I repeatedly encounter this truth about how physical energy relates to mental health, it always comes as a surprise. In fact, I recently discovered that denying the physical frailties in my post-cancer life can be as dangerous as the cancer.

When the fall semester ended, I tucked my last batch of

papers into my suitcase and, with Noel and two friends, flew south to Mexico and learned a lesson. The idea was for me to sit under the shade of my hat brim and dry out my lungs. My brother-in-law, Ken, and his companion had arranged for a place on the Baja outside San Jose de Cabos where a visitor can fall asleep to the sound of breakers the size of a wall. The first night I stood on our balcony listening to the surf and breathing in the warm dry air. Stars filled the night with magic, and an endless beach made me dream of the next day.

By dawn the sands had become reddish gold with the rising sun. Palm trees patterned my view of the aquamarine water. After breakfast and grading papers, I wandered along the beach and watched Ken dive through a big wave. It looked inviting and I followed him, swimming under the surf to a calm place where I surfaced for air. A foreign noise between a kettle whistling and a goose honking came out of my mouth as I tried to catch my breath, and I learned the palpable meaning of the word *suffocate*. After using an oxygen tank on the airplane to ensure that the pressure change and the recycled air caused me no pulmonary distress, I had not considered the pressure of water against my less flexible lung. Pulmonary fibrosis, a growing crinkle of scar tissue from my chemotherapy and radiation, had left me with less bargaining power against the Pacific Ocean. Unable to breathe, I heard Ken, keeping me afloat, coax me not to turn my back on the big wave that would hit as we rode it to shore. I hissed that I had staples holding my front ribs together. I meant it as a joke, but his expression was grim. Doing a sort of sidestroke, I clung to his shoulder. By this time Noel had recognized the problem from shore and was there to lift me into the air and through the wave.

I have become a stranger to the person who used to swim

thoughtlessly with these same arms and legs, but with a different pair of bellows. I saw the look on Noel's face, our mirrored recognition of my inability to inhale enough air. I laughed through my gasps and coughing when the water deposited us on the beach. Remembering the many times I had taken myself to the water's edge without fear, I realized this day marked a new awareness. My independence had been diminished, but it had been replaced by a gratitude that swelled with the waves that separated me from my companions.

As I waited for the men to return, I cleared my thoughts by reading the washing instructions printed on the label inside my hat: *any river or creek will do.* Oceans are in another league from rivers and creeks – salt on the wound of a ravaged lung. I thought about early Canadian poems and stories I have shared with students, tales of settlers forced to recognize nature's power and of man's foolish pride in trying to tamper with its supremacy. I too am an explorer, however minor, in a land where everything physical has new dimensions, surprising ones, but surmountable within a redefined set of boundaries.

And this perhaps is my secret to living with cancer, the story I have to tell myself again and again. My old life has ended and my new life has established itself. Such is the power of this disease. It surpasses all else in its immediacy, its need for recognition. This is the story that all cancer patients must tell themselves. The *terra firma* has changed; the solid earth has new areas of quicksand. I live now in *terra incognita*, an unknown land, at least until I learn more about the renovated house where my spirit dwells. The warm Pacific taught me, regardless of metastasis, I am just a heartbeat away from death if I neglect the frailties of the flesh. In the warm winds of the Baja, I learned again to take nothing for granted.

My attempts to express a truth about hope would not be balanced if I did not confess to fear and sorrow. I am tinged with sorrow from the loss of family, friends, and illusions of immortality. But this is true of everyone who reaches middle age, of course, not just cancer patients. Some days my mother's eyes look into mine from somewhere in the register of memory: I see her busy over an evening meal, musing about a grandchild's having emptied the raisin jar or an unusual bird she saw in her garden. Sometimes I hear a sigh escape my lips and realize I have caught a memory of my father's thick white hair, his slowing gait, and the green eyes that suggested a wistful longing once my mother was gone. Sometimes I glimpse the face of Joyce, or Skip, or Kathleen in the crowd. These moments sustain my stash of precious memories, the fulfillment of the past, their support of me now.

I can bolster myself too by contemplating obvious signs of progress in my health. Skiing, for example, tells a story of change. On my first visit to Whistler after my diagnosis and before my treatments, pneumonia held me captive, shivering and sweating. I tossed and turned on the Murphy bed Noel had installed to give us more room in our tiny home on the hill. He went off to ski with friends, and I comforted myself that one of these friends, a cardiologist, could help me if my health suddenly deteriorated. She too had encouraged me to reserve my energy for the days ahead. After the three of them left to ski, I phoned my respirologist. He advised me to return to Victoria in case an opening came up at the cancer clinic and I could hasten my first visit. As I hung up, Noel came through the door, confessing that he couldn't enjoy himself skiing while I lay ill in the lodge. We packed our bags.

A year later, after my treatments, we went again to Whistler. I had recently been diagnosed with the shingles, and another doctor had told me I might not be able to breathe at altitude. He assured me, however, that the worst thing that would happen is that I might faint. I barely noticed the thinning oxygen, except for the hot air that Noel expelled when I told him, in the gondola, that I might faint from dizziness. I skied down twice in one day before my body complained too loudly to ignore. Then, in 1996, a new confidence invaded my spirit in spite of Whistler's blizzard winds and record cold temperatures. I managed two long runs on separate days before my energy bottomed out. These gifts of change told me that my treatments have been worthwhile and that my complementary therapies encourage my body to thrive.

My elation was dampened, however, when the past came back to haunt me. At the long wooden table in the lodge where we sipped our tea and shared a muffin, a man chatted with his two children. As he helped his daughter and son with their cumbersome boots and jackets, the boy looked up into his father's eyes. I could hear him telling his father of his bravery on the last run. In that single gesture, I relived the one wound that, for me, is greater than any cancer could be – the reminder that I will never look into the eyes of my own child and will never know the reason for being denied this profound privilege. But even here cancer has changed me. I no longer take a swift breath and look away. Instead, I bide with my sorrow a while, look it in the eye, and eventually feel the hollow fill with the joys I have now. I have learned that the light of life is always brighter when it contrasts the darkness.

Vulnerable, exuberant, grateful – these words describe my feelings during this precious time of remission. Having completed the journey from limbo to love, from horror to hope, I am no longer as anxious as I once was. Lost however is the pre-cancerous sense of invulnerability. Fear enters my life when I drive a rain-slicked highway, feel an airplane take off, or kayak in heavy currents. I see danger where there is none and seek safety more often than before. Cancer has taught me to safeguard myself from carcinogens and from my genetic susceptibility to disease, and to seek health by nestling deep within the arms of joy and thankfulness.

Some cancer patients, I realize, are not well enough to see their dreams into experience, as I have done in writing this book, remarrying, vacationing in Italy and Mexico, and buying a puppy. Some patients have to find courage to struggle alone, not having the support of an imaginative partner. The stamina demanded of these patients should not pass unnoticed. Each day they create miracles through perseverence and dignity, some with access to nothing but their own deep wells of determination. These people are heroes who have done alone what I have done with the help of others. Some hide their wounds behind a face of courage. Others are forced to share the embarrassment of newly lost hair, surgical scars, and weight loss. These are people who find comfort in the small kindnesses of strangers, in the charity of action, and in the compassion of recognition.

Perhaps some patients would gain from the gift of an appointment with an alternative therapist instead of flowers, books, or fruit. Not everyone can afford complementary treatments even though their cost is small compared to traditional medicine. Alternative therapies are rarely covered by medical insurance and then only in limited measure. When I heard a highly paid specialist on the radio criticizing people for paying therapists fees for their services, I wondered if he realized that this fee is approximately what a medical doctor charges to fill in forms for disability insurance. An imbalance needs to be rectified here, in response to public demand. The combined voice of patients is spreading the need to link modern means with ancient ways that cannot be measured by scientific rules alone.

Frustrating too are those moments when even my tentative sense of control vanishes. My medical appointments remind me that I am in remission. However slowly the clock ticks, the appointment comes too slowly and too quickly. I want the answer immediately and never. I am a living question mark. Doctors and patients alike wait in ignorance for laboratory results. As I wait, I know that one succinct word rolling off the doctor's tongue could change the world for me again. I have to steel myself to maintain my view that statistics do not account for the unique, a definition I apply to myself. I use this argument of uniqueness when Noel refuses me a second glass of wine on a Friday night.

And then there is the hour of the wolf, the truth that comes just before dawn. Some call these moments panic attacks, but I prefer Ingmar Bergman's expression. I have not yet had to hear the bad news of cancer twice, but the idea punches me in the solar plexus when I awaken to darkness. Heidi, my chemotherapist, stood beside me in January 1997 as she put my new x-rays onto the lighted screen. *Oh dear,* she said, and my world collapsed. At that moment I could not remember the word *unique,* only that a recurrence of a primary cancer in the lung is highly likely. Heidi explained that she had forgotten to bring in last summer's x-rays for comparison. As she left the room, my stomach unclenched and my limbs turned to custard. I could hear myself recapturing my breath.

When she returned I told her about my new puppy. Through

a smile, she promised she would phone me with the results and said my new x-ray looked good. The speckled light between the end of one day and the dawn of the next seemed to last a century. If I had not had the good fortune of connecting with a compassionate oncologist, I may have waited a week or two to discover that I had yet again avoided death row. With my reprieve, I suffer from the exhaustion of overwhelming relief.

The hour of the wolf took on a second meaning when I read a newspaper story about a wolf that became a metaphor for human possibility, a four-legged Houdini. This wolf had defied scientific absolutes, as cancer patients wish to do, even though it had lost half its jaw in a battle with a wolf of the opposite sex. To save the animal from a slow death by starvation, the zoo keepers and veterinarians had injected a powerful cocktail into its broken heart. They put its body in the morgue freezer and left it there until morning, when they gathered to do an autopsy. Once the animal was returned to the operating table, it struggled to its feet, shook itself off, and walked away. Since people respond well to proof that the living spirit can stretch to inspirational heights, the veterinarians named him Lazarus for his miraculous return to life and combined their energies to build him a new jaw. Lazarus was last seen by his admirers slurping up mashed food.

Just as an impossibly happy ending makes cancer patients rejoice, skeptics make it hard for those who live under threat of the surgeon's knife or, worse, beyond the help of surgery. Just as one patient's courage makes others follow, one sympathetic ear teaches another. But even at the end of the twentieth century, some people cannot hear the word *cancer* spoken aloud, so great is their fear, so intense their subjective reaction. I have known someone to call me *jinxed* to avoid the connectedness that compassion implies, and someone else to stop kissing me on the cheek in case cancer is contagious. These are the rotten apples I discard before they can destroy the solid flesh and rosy cheek of hope.

Lorna Crozier wrote a series of poems entitled *Everything Arrives at the Light*. Her poems explore the idea that shadows distinguish the spiritual and intellectual illumination waiting for those who seek its clarity. I leave the dark behind each time I dance into this promised light. It explodes in a kaleidoscope of shimmering possibilities.

This book is set in Bembo, a typeface produced by
Stanley Morison of Monotype in 1929.
Bembo is based on a roman typeface cut by Francesco
Griffo in 1495; the companion italic is based on
a font designed by Giovanni Tagliente in the 1520s.

Book design and typesetting by
James Ireland Design Inc., Toronto